Setting the Stage

Setting the Stage

Delivering the Plan Using the Learner's Brain Model

Dr. Mario C. Barbiere

ROWMAN & LITTLEFIELD
Lanham • Boulder • New York • London

Published by Rowman & Littlefield
A wholly owned subsidiary of The Rowman & Littlefield Publishing Group, Inc.
4501 Forbes Boulevard, Suite 200, Lanham, Maryland 20706
www.rowman.com

Unit A, Whitacre Mews, 26–34 Stannary Street, London SE11 4AB

British Library Cataloguing in Publication Information Available

Library of Congress Cataloging-in-Publication Data Is Available
Names: Barbiere, Mario C., author.
Title: Setting the stage : delivering the plan using the learner's brain model /
    Mario C. Barbiere.
Description: Lanham, Maryland : Rowman & Littlefield, 2018. | Includes
    bibliographical references.
Identifiers: LCCN 2018016076 (print) | LCCN 2018002285 (ebook) |
    ISBN 9781475837247 (cloth : alk. paper) | ISBN 9781475837230
    (pbk. : alk. paper) | ISBN 9781475837254 (electronic)
Subjects: LCSH: Learning, Psychology of. | Learning—Physiological aspects. | Brain.
Classification: LCC LB1060 .B373 2018 (ebook) | LCC LB1060 (print) |
    DDC 370.15/23—dc23
LC record available at https://lccn.loc.gov/2018016076

♾️™ The paper used in this publication meets the minimum requirements of American National Standard for Information Sciences—Permanence of Paper for Printed Library Materials, ANSI/NISO Z39.48–1992.

Printed in the United States of America

This book is dedicated to my wife Alice, who always believed in me. Her wisdom, kindness, and compassion will always be remembered. A former teacher and mother who inspired students, children, and grandchildren.

It is also dedicated to Jim and Mairin, Kaleb, Kaia; Chris; Mike and Jackie, and Matt. Her spirit lives on in our hearts.

Contents

Preface

After decades of experience in education and working with many teachers and educators, I decided to develop rubrics for teachers and administrators, which can be used for self-improvement or for administrators to use for coaching teachers. The initial rubrics were well received, so I continued to develop rubrics for all phases of instructional delivery. Prior to working on the rubric, I had spent ten years studying brain research leading to my doctoral dissertation on brain research and lesson design. I decided to marry the work I had done on brain research with the work on rubrics.

During the time I was doing research for this book, I was working as a Network Turnaround Officer (NTO) involved in school turnaround. NTOs were hired to work in low-performing schools as part of a School Improvement Grant (SIG), which New Jersey received. This job began a new phase of my educational career path. The work became a driving passion for me.

School turnaround is not just focusing on low-performing schools but focusing on all children and closing achievement gaps as well. It represents providing hope for all, so the work is extremely important as educators never want to extinguish a student's hope or dreams.

The teachers and administrators found the rubrics helpful in providing targeted feedback. The feedback from the rubrics provided encouragement for the book. This book is written beginning with understanding the nature of the learner so lessons can be effectively planned. Following the nature of the learner, the reader is provided suggestions for planning the lesson. After the lesson is planned, a Readiness Set is used to begin the instruction. The final chapter discusses making sense and meaning for promoting long-term memory.

Please enjoy this book, and your comments are welcome.

Acknowledgments

As a teacher, vice principal, principal, assistant superintendent, and superintendent I have had the opportunity to work with many talented and caring educators at all levels of education, and their commitment to educating children is acknowledged and appreciated.

A special thank you to the Roosevelt School, South Plainfield, New Jersey, teachers and staff during the years 1978–2003 whose hard work and dedication made student believers, education stimulating, and twenty-five years of administration rewarding. Pat Hajduk, Sharon Padula, and Adele Viers made coming to work enjoyable, especially during the challenging times.

Bill Andersen, Dr. Fran Borkes, Dr. JoAnn Berkley, Neyda Evans, Kate Gallagher, Sheila Wegryn, and Frank Zalocki, with whom I had the opportunity to work with doing school turnaround with great success, provided years of friendship, meaningful work, and success. Thanks team—we had a lot of laughs, great memories, and great successes.

Thank you to Jane Wiatr for her suggestions, editing, and advice.

Thank you to Carlie Wall, managing editor, Rowman & Littlefield, for her suggestions and input.

A special thanks to Rowman & Littlefield, especially Tom Koerner, for helping a dream become a reality.

Introduction

This book is designed for the teachers or administrators to use for planning lessons. Unlike other texts that focus on planning, this text focuses on developing lessons knowing the nature of the learner. This book does not attempt to "change" the teacher but instead focuses on the learner so the teacher can adapt his or her lessons based on the nature of the learner. Knowing the nature of the learner will allow teachers to plan engaging activities and lessons.

After the nature of the learner is introduced, chapter 2 presents the Learner's Brain Model. This chapter begins unpacking the Learner's Brain Model. The first step of the model is planning/readiness and establishing the learning domain. The role of climate, environment emotional security, mood, and classroom management are parts of the model that will be addressed.

Chapter 2 defines the following areas of lesson design for the Learner's Brain Model: planning, instruction, establishing the domain, developing the Essential Question, planning the Student Learning Target (SLT) (objective), and assessing the target via a Teacher Assessment of Learning, or "Demonstration of Student Learning," which is referred to throughout this book as a DSL. The planning stage is necessary for the delivery of coherent instruction. Once the planning is determined, how the instruction is to be delivered is the next chapter.

Chapter 3 helps educators to develop a Readiness Set to get the student's interest at the onset of a lesson or at the beginning of a new lesson. After the Readiness Set, the teacher plans the lesson to "make sense" and have meaning for the student. This phase is Stage 1 of the Readiness Cycle.

To get the student interests, the Readiness Set has three components: the starter (also called a catalyst, hook, or attention getter), the connection of what will be taught to what students know, and the tie in of the new information to the students' prior knowledge. Once the student interest is hooked, the next task is for the teacher to implement a lesson that makes sense and has meaning to the student.

The development of sense and meaning begins the next phase of the Learner's Brain Model: the informational stage. The informational stage involves providing teacher-directed instruction, student-directed instruction, independent work, small group activities, and/or cooperative activities. Strategies for each phase of the informational stage will be provided.

The Learner's Brain Model uses right and left brain research for lesson design, which makes sense (logical) part of the brain and makes sense (global). Lessons need the logical (left brain) and the global perspective (right brain) to move from the "informational" age to the "conceptual" age. To move to that phase, lessons must apply information and concepts to real-life problems.

In summary, the text begins with understanding the nature of the learner, planning a lesson based on how the learner learns, using a Readiness Set to get the students interested, and finally applying the learning to real-life problems as the information makes sense and has meaning.

Chapter 1

The Nature of the Learner

FOCUS OF THE CHAPTER

What is the nature of the learner? How can teachers plan lessons to promote long-term learning and student self-regulation?

INTRODUCTION

The question "what is the nature of the learner?" has been asked time and time again. Understanding the nature of the learner allows teachers to construct effective instruction and promote student self-regulation. This chapter introduces a model for lesson design and instruction based on understanding the nature of the learner.

Probing Questions

1. How can teachers use brain research to design lessons to meet student needs?
2. How can knowing how students learn be used for lesson planning?
3. How can educators help students self-regulate their learning?

THE LEARNER'S BRAIN MODEL

This book addresses the question of how teachers can plan lessons using the Learner's Brain Model and how students can self-regulate their learning to become more self-dependent and not teacher-dependent.

The four stages of the Learner's Brain Model consists of the planning stage, the readiness stage, the informational stage, and the consolidaton stage. Each stage will be described in detail throughout this book. The chapters will address how the teacher can execute the stage and what the student must do to self-regulate. Since the end product is the student, we will start by understanding the nature of the learner so we know the framework to use to develop lessons to meet their needs.

BACKGROUND: BRAIN RESEARCH LEADS THE PATH TO STUDYING

The Nature of the Learner

When thinking about studying brains, one would ponder, "What better brain to study than Einstein's brain?" Dr. Thomas Harvey removed Einstein's brain shortly after his death in 1955 for the purpose of scientific research. Three years later, Dr. Harvey lamented that nothing was published about the results of the study of Einstein's brain so the brain went back to the jar of formaldehyde where it was kept in a box under a beer cooler in Harvey's office. It would be many more years before researchers had the opportunity to use brain research techniques and instruments to study the nature of the learner.

Welcome Federal Government

The impetus for brain research would get a push from a congressional proclamation in 1989. New curricula would focus on the learner's brain or brain research.

Because the development of new curricula was a risky economic venture, commercial developers decided to leave it to the federal government to provide financial support. Once the federal government began to support such programs, a process was established that began with scholars at the university level and filtered down to teachers at the local level. The federal government would invest millions in curriculum projects.

The Federal Government's Working Assumptions

A set of working assumptions formed the basis of the approach of the National Science Foundation (NSF) to implementation. Programs would focus on the quality of science education among schools, not on directly increasing scientific and technical manpower. NSF interviews would be integrative rather than programmatic. Funds would not be directed to students in classrooms but to intermediate points of entry in the educational system because of budget limitations and NSF staffers' convictions that this would be more effective in the long run.

The Federal Government Invests in Curriculum

Funds would not be used to create programs administered by the government but to provide activities designed to bring together personnel who would not ordinarily be involved in educational improvement activities. Consequently, the NSF projects involved teachers and other specialists including scientists, discipline and curriculum experts, university professors, and educators; they influenced school curricula by funding conferences, projects, teacher training institutes, and curriculum writers.

The Decade of the Brain

The 1990s saw significant change in focus from curriculum to brain research. With the advent of technology, researchers were able to better understand how the human brain collects, processes, and interprets information. President George H. W. Bush's declaration that the 1990s was the "Decade of the Brain" was prescient and insightful. The president predicted that a new era of discovery was dawning in brain research as a result of an explosion of information on how the brain works.

The decade saw numerous research projects and the development and use of the position emission tomography (PET) scan to assess how a learner learns. It also saw television programs, books, and magazine articles that offered simplistic comments concerning how to "improve" memory. Brain research was moving at a fast rate.

From Brain Research to Brain Bandwagon

Nowadays, before educators can jump 100 percent on the brain research bandwagon, they need to better understand how the brain learns and how to use that knowledge to prepare lessons designed to maximize learning. Functional magnetic resonance imaging (fMRI) and PET scans, for example, offer insight into brain functioning by producing three-dimensional maps of the human brain that allow researchers to plot those areas of the brain that are stimulated when learning takes place. The tests describe what happens in the learner's brain which makes it easier for teachers to design their lessons based on the nature of the learner.

It is generally agreed that teachers need to address learners' emotions, connect learning activities to learners' experiences, engage the learners via a multisensory approach using two or more senses, and design "shorter les-sons" so students are not sitting and listening to a teacher lecture but are actively involved in the learning process. Of particular importance was early childhood education and early second-language instruction to enable students to start to build their knowledge base.

Brain Bandwagon Begins with Early Childhood Education

The need for early childhood education for two to four year olds is important because children are born with an estimated 12 to 15 billion nerve cells (neu-rons). Each neuron interacts with other neurons by extending branches (den-drites). What brain researchers discovered was that the number of synapses per unit volume of tissue (called synaptic density) changes over a person's life span. Infants are born with more brain cells than they need.

By age four, their synaptic densities are 50 percent higher than that of an adult. By puberty, a pruning process begins by eliminating synapses that are not used and myelinating the neurons that are used. Hence the adage, "Use it or lose it."

If children are born with more synapses than necessary, questions arise as to what happens to the extra ones, whether extra-synaptic densities mean that certain individuals are more intelligent than others, and whether there is a direct relationship between synaptic densities and intelligence.

Some research suggests that neuroscience research demonstrated no direct relationship between synaptic densities and intelligence as the changes in the synaptic densities resembled an inverted-U pattern with the representation being high at birth and childhood and lower in adulthood.

Plasticity Factor

More researchers now believe in the "plasticity factor" of the brain to dispute the old theory that the brain is "hard-wired" and that a child's intelligence is fixed at birth. We now believe that the brain's ability to constantly change its structure and function in response to experience coming in from the outside leads to the concept of learning as being dynamic as opposed to static.

Since children are born with more brain cells than they need, and as a result of "pruning," some brain cells survive and some perish; brain cells that are stimulated survive. It is also important, therefore, that learning experiences involve the several senses (vision, hearing, smell, touch, and taste) as information is stored in various parts of the brain from the sensory input. When teachers want to ensure that information goes into long-term memory, we ask, "How do we go from 'first messenger' or sensory input to deeper learning?"

In order to ensure that information is processed in the brain, the synapses must be stimulated so that connections become part of the structure that is retained. Making new connections is what is known as "learning."

The Learning Environment

An important factor impacting learning is the environment that is established. In the learning environment, informational charts, anchor charts, rubrics, and exemplars all help students self-regulate their learning. This way, they can self-manage and self-monitor their progress, facilitated by an enriched learning environment. Learners who are engaged in a rich learning environment will also have an effective result with an increase in the intelligence quotient (IQ) scores.

Research done by Diamond (1998) focused on how the brain changes physically in response to environment. She investigated the changes in the cerebral cortex, the quarter-inch thick blanket of cells that covers the brain. In one experiment, she investigated the changes in the cerebral cortex when rats were exposed to two different environments.

Rats in the experimental group interacted with an "enriched environment" that included toys and other objects for exploration and climbing. Rats in the control group lived in an "impoverished" environment. Diamond observed that the rats in the "enriched" environment developed a thicker cortex than those living in the "impoverished" environment (1998).

The nerve cells in the brains of the rats in the experimental group were stimulated, and their cortexes manifested new cell growth. Their cells were stimulated and new dendrites, the receptive surface of the cell, were formed. The receptors and number of connections among the cells were increased.

Long-lasting functional changes (plasticity) occurred in the brains of the experimental rats in direct response to their experiences in the "enriched" environment. The larger question to explore is, does the change last or is it just a short-term gain that fades over time?

Moving from Short-Term Learning to Long-Term Learning

As educators, we are all familiar with the effects of short-term learning in which the teacher prepares students before a test. They take the test and do well but after a day, the learning dissipates. We are well aware of folks who studied for a test the night before (or "cramming" as it is called) for the test, and a few days later forget everything.

As teachers, however, we want the short-term learning to go into long-term memory. One way to get information to long-term memory is by applying the skills and concepts being taught into a performance task. When we teach for competency, students will know facts, figures, and procedural information and are able to solve a problem, but may not be able to translate those problem-solving skills when faced with real-life situations.

If we are teaching for performance, we are asking students to apply facts, figures, and information. Performance automatically begets competency because students are applying the skills learned. However, competency doesn't automatically get performance.

Educators see the shift from competency to performance in our state assessments. Students are asked to know and apply what they learn. The shift to application from competency is seen with the Partnership for Assessment Readiness for College and Career (PARCC) tests as they are considered to be more rigorous. Teachers require students to apply what is that they know. The push for real-life application is not only more rigorous, but it also helps the students to see how learning will be applied in the real world.

Finding "Meaning" and Purpose

While an enriched learning environment has an impact on how students learn, what students do in the environment has a direct impact on knowledge retention. A critical factor in knowledge acquisition is helping students find "meaning" and purpose in classroom activities, or learning does not take place. Retention does not occur beyond the classroom door if the lesson lacks sense and meaning. Retention may not even occur within the classroom if the lesson does not make sense or have meaning.

Developing Sense and Meaning

The value of developing meaning and helping students make sense is critical. As teachers, we know right away if students have internalized the learning if they ask the killer questions: Why are we learning this? Will this information going to be on the test? What the student is saying is that the information has no value or meaning, but "if it is on a test or quiz, I will try to understand." In these scenarios, the students lack a reason for learning the material. If they do learn it, they will probably forget it right after the test.

Imagine a scenario whereby the "killer questions" are asked and the teacher responds in a different manner. For the "why do we have to learn this" question, the teacher can give the student several applications and activities to do so that students can see how the information can be applied. The activities should involve real-life tasks so the need for the information becomes transparent.

Gradual Release to Develop Sense and Meaning

Another technique for developing sense and meaning is to use a delivery method called gradual release. The teacher releases the learner by a three-step approach: I do, we do, and you do.

For math, and to help students discover meaning, the process can be reversed: you do, we do, and I do. The "you do" begins by having students presented with a problem to do. They work in small groups to discuss the problem and use math vocabulary to solve it. This approach allows the student to work on the problem, use productive struggle to solve the problem, and then develop questions to ask the teacher.

The need for skills to solve the problem becomes evident when the students are working on problems which help them understand the need for skill development. After the student experiences some frustration, the teacher can do a "we do" activity. At this stage the student would be more receptive to learning skills because they need the information to solve the problem. The final stage for the process is the teacher's "I do" stage where the teacher models the learning and talks about strategies during the modeling demonstration.

Teacher modeling of lessons for the students while explaining his or her thinking throughout the process helps the student to develop self-regulation skills. The modeling is also important for developing self-regulation skills, as students will now be working with partners and sharing their thinking.

Using the Learning Environment to Promote Self-Regulation

The teacher can remind the learners that if they are having any difficulty or are stuck, they can use the information to help them because the classroom is "environmentally constructed," that is, there are rubrics, exemplars, informational charts to enhance student self-regulation. The teacher can also help promote self-regulation by reminding the students to seek out other resources before going to the teacher for help. This is sometimes called "two before me." They can ask a friend or use the resources in the room, or they can use the Internet prior to going to the teacher or friend.

Using Home Learning

The teacher can also give a home learning assignment in which the students write in their journals to reflect on their learning and how they arrived at their answer. The teacher can then review the student's journal and provide feedback so as to help the student promote self-regulation and promote metacognition.

Journaling will help develop student metacognition because students will be thinking about the problem and seeking ways to solve it. If during a review, the teacher sees that students are very cryptic in their response, the teacher can make a list of questions for the students to answer. The questions can promote metacognition if the students are asked to explain, justify, or rationalize their answers. (Later in this book we will discuss the value of feedback and questioning.)

The Value of Journaling

Another value of journaling is that the language arts teacher can be involved in helping students journal, take notes, or develop effective writing skills. With the new PARCC, there are standards that are integrated, so that science and social studies teachers can integrate their assignments and activities with language arts teachers. PARCC has "integrated" standards, identified as "INT." An integrated standard is one that is integrated across content areas or within a grade/course.

When we look at PARCC questions that have a reading and science or social studies component, we see students getting information from a video or from reading from multiple sources. For science, it is more than doing an experiment but reading the research associated the experiment then explain the research.

The approach for PARCC is different from just doing the experiment, because the experiment shows competency of the scientific method. Reading about the experiment includes reasoning and higher levels of cognition of synthesis and analysis.

Making New Connections

Tying in new knowledge to previous knowledge allows new connections to be formed. As information gets used, it moves from short-term to long-term memory. The second time the neurons fire they become more efficient and interactions fire more easily.

It is important to remember that no two learners are alike and they may respond differently to an enriched learning environment. Teachers should deliver lessons that incorporate various learning styles. More importantly, teachers need to teach self-regulation skills to students in order for them to be self-dependent and not teacher-dependent.

Brain-based research and research on how children learn make clear that the brain changes physiologically as a result of experience. The environment in which the brain operates determines to a large degree the functioning ability of that brain. The environment affects nerve cells; nerve cells interpret the environment. When nerve cells respond to the environment, dendrites grow. When they are appropriately stimulated, new dendrites grow.

Home Environment versus Learning Environment

When talking about the learning environment, teachers are apt to talk about the home environment as opposed to the classroom environment. It is important to remember that teachers have a locus of control that is the classroom and not the home environment. In the classroom, the playing field is leveled for all students because there will be opportunities provided to students, regardless of their family or home environment.

To claim that a student will not do well because of the family or home environment dooms a child to failure. Certainly, an enriched home environment is a plus; however, for students who do not have that luxury, teachers have to provide a supportive and enriched environment in the classroom. The teacher needs to focus on working with the variables that he or she can control, that is, the classroom and not the factors that are out of his or her control.

Teachers Compensate for a Poor Home Environment

Teachers' focus on those things that cannot be controlled will only lead to frustration and other concerns, and will give ammunition for teachers to have excuses as to why the students cannot do well in school. The teachers' focus should be on ensuring that the learning environment is adaptable for all students so that teachers do not have a "one-size-fits-all model."

The one-size-fits-all model is basically teaching to the middle group. When teachers teach to the middle group, the high group is bored and the low group will need more time. It is better to give all students what they need.

Providing Need and Not Want: Equity versus Equality

If one has $10 and two children who need money, in order to be equal one would give each child $5. Let's say that one child has $7 and needs $3 to make $10 and the other has $3 and needs $7 to make $10. If each child gets $5 the one with $3 will have $8 or $2 less than what is needed and the one with $7 would have $12 or $2 more than what is needed.

People should get what they need. Teachers should plan to differentiate the lessons based on tiered activities, giving students what they need as opposed to giving all students the same.

BRAIN FACTS AND THE ENVIRONMENT

In the Beginning

Dewey (1938) wrote about the importance of environment and the experience in the environment relative to the construction of curriculum. He wrote that it is not enough to insist upon the necessity of experience, but the quality of the activity planned in the experience. The quality of the experience is important because experience for the sake of experience does not ensure that children learn. Learning is more than providing experience and expecting knowledge. Cognitive activity must be purposeful and directed, not inferential and aimless.

Contemporary brain-based research insists on the need for a planned, controlled environment that provides meaningful experiences that are beneficial to children and promote self-regulation. When we permit chance environments to do the work, or whether we design and construct environments with a purpose, it makes a great difference between success and failure.

One finds in the contemporary work of Sousa, Wolfe, Brandt, and Kotulak echoing the advice given by Dewey in many of his works but notably in *Experience and Education* (1938) and *Democracy and Education* (1916).

IQ Is Not Fixed at Birth

Brain research makes clear that IQ is not fixed at birth. Ramey and Ramey (1996) built on previous research and tested the findings on the impact of environment on brain cell growth in rats and their implications for human brain cell growth. Ramey and Ramey directed various studies that included thousands of children. Their purpose was to determine if infants' scores on intelligence tests could be raised by manipulating the environment in ways similar to Diamond's manipulation of the rats' environment.

Ramey and Ramey's data demonstrated that the children's scores on intelligence tests were raised by 15 to 30 percent. Their data sampled children whose ages ranged from six weeks to four months. They concluded that being at risk did not mean that the students were doomed. Indeed, it is the teacher who can and will make a critical difference to each student.

Value of Early Educational Experiences

Educators know that when it comes to brain research relative to young children, the value of early educational experiences is important.

Marion Diamond (1998), a researcher who studied anatomy and physiology of the brain for more than forty years, was interviewed on how the brain changes physically in response to the environment. The researcher questioned her about working with animals because of the similar structure and behavior of nerve cells across species. Diamond (1998) explained that she likes working with rats as there were no human being who volunteered their cerebral cortes. In her studies she found that rats living in and enriched environment.

Obviously, the results of the research conducted by Diamond on enriched environments speak of the enhancement of brain cell growth in an enriched environment.

The results were also not limited to impoverished children but to other groups. To test the work of Ramey and Ramey (and Greenough), Jeanne Brooks-Gunn of Columbia University's Teachers College, New York, studied premature infants (approximately 1,000 infants) at various centers. The ten centers that were used reported that the intervention group had significantly higher IQs than infants in the control group.

The question becomes, then, did the intellectual benefits last? The concern may be that interventions were applied, but were they short term or a "flash in the pan."

Early Childhood Education and Federal Legislation

Evidently, the benefits of early intervention are not going to be overlooked, as with the new federal legislation of No Child Left Behind (2000), more and more research is required to receive federal funding for programs. In addition to early interventions and enriched environments, the role of emotions is critical in the learning process.

Whether one calls the activity "downshifting," or "cooling down," it is clear that emotions have a significant part in the educational process.

EMOTIONS

Emotions Drive Learning

Emotions drive everything. Student learning has an emotional component that drives their willingness to learn. We can all remember a negative experience and can think back to high school's days of pleasurable and negative experiences. We remember the positive experiences because of the emotional attachment to the experience, and we try to extinguish the negative experience. We are more inclined to seek resolution to problems that have an emotional attachment.

What becomes critical then is for the teacher to understand how significant emotions are in the educational process. Another consideration is ensuring that students are also in touch with their emotions since emotions are part of an unconscious arousal system.

Having a safe and orderly school environment, as well as students cognizant of stress reduction, conflict management, and biofeedback, helps to ensure emotional security. Students who do not have a conscious understanding of their emotional state often do foolish things.

It is important to help students understand how emotions and feelings affect behavior. A student will do something foolish and when questioned why he or she did that, the student may often reply: "I don't know." Their emotions overrule their rational thinking. It is therefore necessary for teachers to teach students strategies for self-control, and how to self-regulate, self-manage, and self-monitor their learning so they become empowered and not enabled.

Emotional Intelligence

Various authors, including Daniel Goldman, have written about emotional intelligence. It wasn't until technology was able to catch up with Goleman's theory, with the help of Joseph LeDoux (1994, 1996, 2000, 2002), a neuroscientist at the Center for Neural Science at New York University, that his theory could be proven. Neural pathways were pinpointed, and LeDoux discovered that information entering through the senses of vision and hearing initially went to the thalamus. If the information was emotional, the thalamus sent out responses to two parts of the brain.

The emotional brain has the information first, and in the event of a crisis it can react before the thinking brain has even received the information and has had a chance to weigh the options and determine what to do. Since the brain is concerned about our survival, having the unconscious ability for fight or flight will allow us minimum time if making a decision.

From Intake to Long-Term Memory

Once the information is taken in, how do we move the information to long-term memory from the sensory intake stage? The process starts with constructing levels or skills from a single unit. The next step is to expand the single units by "mapping" or having the single unit connect to previous units, which is like "hugging." The single unit needs a "bro hug," or an attachment to other units and multiple units is formed. The multiple units are joined into systems; after a system is developed, the next level begins.

Educators should keep the following in mind:

- The cyclical nature of cortical growth and optimal cognitive development is that there can be continuous growth because the neural connections are "plastic' and not hard-wired. The adage is that we are never too old to learn.
- Brain development involves a recurring growth cycle of neural networks and learning.
- Children (and adults) function at multiple levels of skill and understanding.
- An individual's level of skill and understanding depends on high-level functioning so that short-term learning can lead to long-term learning if higher levels of learning are included in the process.
- Educators need to focus on teaching children at all levels as well as on providing differentiated instruction to meet individual needs.

Knowing that cognitive growth and brain growth are linked can lead to a rich and rewarding learning environment, where emotions and age-appropriate activities are included, and that planned, purposeful, and challenging tasks are taken into consideration. All of these require preplanning.

The Role of Learner Interaction

Learning is more than teachers lecturing and students sitting at their desks taking notes. The process is such that learners are involved in activities and interact with their environment. This interaction is important because learners store components of the images they are learning in various parts of their brains.

Items that are similar are stored together. There is storage space for shapes, color, movement, sequence, and textures, for example. The brain makes interwoven connections and stores items in clusters. The critical factor is the quality of the connection and how well the brain organizes and stores the relationships between and among the events' various aspects. Prior knowledge is used to interpret new material, tying the new growth to the old. This helps "orphan information" (new information) get tied to prior information.

Pattern Seeking

Teachers should keep in mind that the student's brain is also a pattern seeker. The brain is always looking for patterns. The planning triangle of interest, prior knowledge, and environment are three considerations that are all interconnected. Having students explore, manipulate, test theories, and predict are all helpful strategies for them to reconstruct their learning as well as bring meaning to the learning.

Written texts are symbols with no reality in the brain's mind's eye, while symbols that have been connected to experience have meaning. A quick test of that concept would be the advertising that is done to help people associate symbols with reality. When someone asks, "Did you BK today?" thoughts of going to a Burger King and eating charbroiled hamburger flash in your mind (assuming you have had prior experience there). If a student is shown a big yellow "M," they would relate it to "McDonalds." These are examples of how our new knowledge is learned by rearranging prior knowledge with new connections.

To further enhance conceptual growth, teachers can incorporate activities that are multisensory and laboratory-oriented, with the knowledge that these projects promote inquiry and activate many areas of the brain. These can range from Full Option Science System (FOSS), Science and Technology for Children, Math in Context to Science Education for Public Understanding

Program. The concept behind these programs is constructivist such that the learners link new knowledge with knowledge already embedded.

Rehearsal Teaching

As teachers approach curriculum development and plan to link old or prior knowledge with the new, they can include concepts like "rehearsal teaching" or practicing the lessons in front of someone else. This concept involves reinforcing what has been learned.

Students can also practice "rehearsal learning." The rehearsal provides knowledge construction and reinforcement, thereby making the concept permanent. The next step is to add something new to the equation so the brain can use the prior knowledge to assimilate the new knowledge, thereby making a connection of the old with the new.

An Example of Rehearsal Teaching

An example of rehearsal teaching is an activity taken from FOSS Balance and Motion module for grades one and two. The first step is for students to balance a cardboard cutout figure on its edge at the tip of the student's finger. The next challenge is to find other ways to balance the cardboard figure, including in-between locations. The balancing and rebalancing of the figure reinforces the students' prior knowledge of what they learned with a new challenge that is slightly different.

An additional challenge is added to find other relations that can develop. Next, mass is added to the cardboard cutout to see how the balance point changes. The rehearsal is when students replicate the task to provide an opportunity to rehearse or practice what was taught.

Rehearsal versus Practice

This notion of rehearsal is different from practice. Practice is repetition of a task to improve the performance of the task. When playing an instrument, the musician will practice scales to improve his or her performance. The practice will involve playing slowing and correctly to learn the scale. The concept of developing speed and proficiency for scales is to "practice slow to get fast." In essence, slow and methodical practice will reinforce proper position and develop muscle memory. Eventually, the practice speed will be increased to the desired level.

Rehearsal, on the other hand, endeavors to promote learning by allowing the brain to recognize that the task that is being learned is not task-specific, but transferable and can be used in a variety of ways, other than only in one particular way. The rehearsals will strengthen the connections among and between the various storage areas. Thus, the adage, "Use it or lose it." To continue with our balancing example, the next logical step is to change the shapes of the figures being used.

Rehearsal provides a student an opportunity to reinforce the learning so various modalities can be used in the practice. The use of manipulatives is a tactile approach. A visual approach includes using pictures, graphs, and the like. The advantage of using multiple sensory systems is useful because information is stored in various areas of the brain. Once information is retrieved, it is like a hologram as information is pulled from the various parts to make a whole picture.

Value of Practice

The value of careful practice is that it gets information into long-term memory. Ask any athlete who has been successful, and they will tell you practice, practice, and practice. Eventually the information goes from short term to long term, and eventually the act becomes second nature.

It is also interesting to note that Dewey expressed his views of tying in the school and society and the child and the curriculum as examples of systems that are integrated.

A Systems Approach—School and Home

Dewey's belief in systems and integration and organic connections is now, 100 years later, the heart of school reform—using a systemic approach to school turnaround. Schools expecting to turnaround have to develop systems, such as systems for attendance, tardiness, chronic absenteeism, and professional development.

It is a systemic plan that ties goals, action plans, and budgets to systems. Systems are the development of sustainable processes. Systems are the key to success, not products. Often the quick fix is sought with the purchase of a product or "one-and-done" programs. Spending money to purchase things for the short term will not get the desired long-term results.

The concept of student achievement is tied to a systems approach as the teacher and student are linked. The approach is for the learning in the classroom to be linked to the real world so students see how theory is tied to practice. Dewey articulated the "link" over 100 years ago.

Instructional Delivery in a "System"

Instructional delivery is also different in a "systems approach" model for teaching. The stand and deliver model will not get the desired results unless the students feel connected to the teacher and the curriculum. Brain research is a valuable link in the instructional process as it provides teachers with information on how students learn.

Brain Research and Instructional Delivery

Following a congressional resolution in 1989, President Bush officially proclaimed the 1990s the "Decade of the Brain." That proclamation was the genesis for explorations on how the brain functions. One wondered: Would educators rush to develop new programming based on the brain research? The short answer is why not? Why not understand the nature of the learner? After all, the end product is the learner, so, as teachers, we need to know our learners and plan our lessons to help them succeed, especially now that we have the technology to determine how the learner is thinking.

The significance of brain research is in applying the findings of brain-based research to instructional delivery for the purpose of creating meaningful and applicable strategies in lesson design.

In conjunction with developing strategies, the educational quandary is to find ways to infuse meaning into what educators teach. Otherwise, punctuating sentences, parsing sentences, measuring angles, solving equations, or analyzing social systems are activities that students' brains will often find meaningless or difficult to understand, and have no value.

Rather than critics of education attacking teachers, let's empower teachers by sharing information with them on how the learner learns so teachers can plan and instruct accordingly. Brain research should be an integral part of teacher training, and added to the knowledge base of how the learner learns, the teacher has all the tools to be successful.

Brain Research, Instructional Delivery, and the Learner's Brain Model

Over the past few years there has been a flood of articles in popular and professional publications discussing the implications of brain science for education and child development. It is important that administrators who consider developing curriculum understand the benefit of brain research tied to how the learner learns so teachers can be more effective in the approach. More importantly, the Learner's Brain Model is presented which incorporates brain research with instructional practices for teachers to use in their instructional delivery.

BIBLIOGRAPHY

Bloom, B. S. 1956. *Taxonomy of Educational Objectives: The Classification of Educational Goals Handbook I: Cognitive Domain.* New York: David McKay Company.

Bookheimer, S. Y., Zeffiro, T. A., Blaxton, T. A., Gaillard , P. W., and Theodore, W. H. 2000. "Activation of Language Cortex with Automatic Speech Tasks." *Neurology* 55(8): 1151–57.

Bush, G. 1990. *Presidential Proclamation 6158.* Library of Congress. http://leweb. loc.gov/loc/brain/proclaim.html.

Cowley, G., and A. Underwood. June 15, 1998. "Memory." *Newsweek* 131 (24): 48–49, 51–54.

Dewey, John. 1895. "The Theory of Emotion (1) Emotional Attitudes." *Psychological Review* 1: 553–69.

———. 1896. "The Reflex Arc Concept in Psychology." *Psychological Review* 3: 357–70.

———. 1902. *The Child and the Curriculum and the School and Society.* Chicago: The University of Chicago Press.

———. 1910. *How We Think.* Lexington, MA: D. C. Heath.

———. 1915. *Schools of Tomorrow.* New York: Dutton Press.

———. 1916. "The Relationship of Thought and Its Subject Matter." In *Essays in Experimental Logic*, 75–102. Chicago: The University of Chicago Press.

———. 1933. *How We Think: A Restatement of the Relation of Reflective Thinking to the Educative Process.* Boston, MA: D. C. Heath & Co Publishers.

———. 1938. *Experience and Education.* New York: Collier Books.

Diamond, M., and J. Hopson. 1998. *Magic Trees of the Mind: How to Nurture Your Child's Intelligence, Creativity and Healthy Emotions from Birth through Adolescence.* New York: Penguin Putnam.

Diamond, M. C., A. B. Scheibel, G. M. Murphy Jr., and T. Harvey. 1985. "On the Brain of a Scientist: Albert Einstein." *Experimental Neurology* 198–204. Retrieved February 18, 2017.

Ebbinghaus, Hermann. 1885. *Memory: A Contribution to Experimental Psychology.* Translated by Henry A. Ruger and Clara E. Bussenino, 1913 edition. New York: Teachers College.

Gazzaniga, M. S., and J. E. LeDoux. 1978. *The Integrated Mind.* New York: Plenum.

Holloway, John. November 2000. "How Does the Brain Learn Science?" *Educational Leadership* 58 (3): 85–86.

Hunter, M. October 1979. "Teaching Is Decision Making." *Educational Leadership* 37(1): 62–64, 67.

———. 1982. *Mastery Teaching.* El Segundo, CA: TIP Publications.

Huttenlocher, P. R., and A. S. Dabholkan. 1997. "Regional Differences in Synaptogenesis in Human Cerebral Cortex." *The Journal of Comparative Neurology* 387: 167–78.

Jensen, Eric. 1998. "How Julie's Brain Learns." *Educational Leadership* 51 (3): 41–46.

Krug, Mark. 1972. *What Will Be Taught: The Nextade*. Itasca, IL: F. E. Peacock Publishers, Inc.

LeDoux, J. E. 1996. *The Emotional Brain*. New York: Simon and Schuster.

———. 1994. "Emotion, Memory and the Brain." *Sci Am* 270: 50–57.

———. 2002. *Synaptic Self: How Our Brains Become Who We Are*. New York: Viking.

———. 2000. "Emotion Circuits in the Brain." *Annu Rev Neurosci* 23: 155–184.

Lepore, F. January 1, 2001. *Dissecting Genius: Einstein's Brain and the Search for the Neural Basis of Intellect*. New York: The Dana Foundation.

Liston, Delores. 1995. "Basic Guidelines for Brain-Compatible Classrooms: Theory to Praxis." Paper presented at the Annual Meeting of the American Education Research Association, San Francisco, CA, April 18–22.

Ramey, C. T., and S. L. Ramey. February 1996. "At Risk Does Not Mean Doomed." *National Health/Education Consortium Occasional Paper, #4*. National Commission to Prevent Infant Morality. Institute for Educational Leadership. Washington, DC.

Sousa, David. 2000. *How the Brain Learns*. Thousand Oaks, CA: Corwin Press.

———. 2001a. *How the Brain Learns, Second Edition*. Thousand Oaks, CA: Corwin Press.

———. 2001b. *How the Special Needs Brain Learns*. Thousand Oaks, CA: Corwin Press.

Wolfe, Pat. 1999. "Revisiting Effective Teaching." *Educational Leadership* 56 (3): 61.

Wolfe, Patricia. 2001. *Brain Matters: Translating Research into Classroom Practice*. Alexandria, VA: Association for Supervision and Curriculum Development.

Chapter 2

Planning Stage for the Learner's Brain Model

FOCUS OF THE CHAPTER

The chapter begins unpacking the Learner's Brain Model. The first step of the model is planning/readiness and establishing the learning domain. The role of climate, environment emotional security, mood, and classroom management are parts of the model that will be addressed.

INTRODUCTION

This chapter will define the following areas of lesson design for the Learner's Brain Model: planning, instruction, establishing the domain, developing the Essential Question, planning the SLT (objective), and assessing the target via Demonstration of Student Learning (DSL).

Probing Questions

1. How do I want scholars to impact my lesson planning?
2. How will I know learning occurred?
3. What are strategies students can use to self-regulate their learning during these phases?

LESSON DESIGN FOR THE LEARNER'S BRAIN MODEL: THE PLANNING STAGE

The first phase of instruction is the planning stage. This stage is specifically geared toward diagnosing the data from the previous lesson as well as the information from the formative assessments and checks for understanding that were conducted. The data will determine what should be taught. It involves learning what needs to be done and how instruction should be implemented and delivered.

OVERVIEW OF THE LEARNER'S BRAIN MODEL

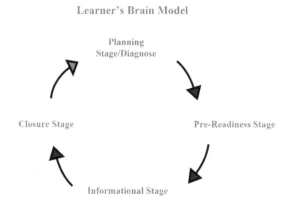

Figure 2.1.

After establishing the first phase and *diagnosing* the data for planning the lesson, the teacher moves to the next phase which is to establish the learning domain or the pre-instructional delivery stage which will be implemented during the lesson.

The Pre-Instruction Delivery Model

While developing the instructional delivery stage, the teacher plans how to create a climate conducive to learning. This climate will provide for social and emotional growth, as well as a safe educational environment in the classroom for the learner.

SETTING THE CLASSROOM ENVIRONMENT

Setting the classroom environment begins with establishing an emotional climate for the instructional cycle. The importance of establishing an emotional climate is rooted in social-emotional learning (SEL) research and is one correlate of an effective school as identified by the research conducted by

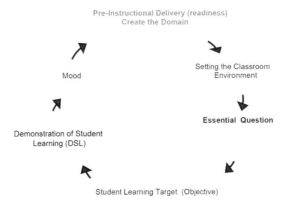

Figure 2.2.

Ron Edmonds for determining effective schools and the research on school turnaround. What was significant about the research on effective schools was that correlates could be applied to any school.

Effective school research has several key characteristics (called correlates) shared by highly effective schools that exist without reference to socioeconomic standards. Students attending schools that exhibit these notable attributes will have a greater chance of academic success, despite the disparity of their home environments. Once applied, the expectation was that there would be high achievement and equitable levels of student learning for all students. These correlates were also included in the principles of school turnaround.

Federal Funds to Promote School Turnaround

Federally funded programs addressing school turnaround were promoted through Race to the Top money. The money could be used for revising teacher evaluations, curriculum development, student tracking systems, or programs to address low-performing schools. School Improvement Grants (SIG) were also made available and the process for school turnaround included turnaround, transformational change, restarting or closing the school.

The Turnaround Process

The process would be guided by eight Turnaround Principles, which are as follows: school leadership; climate and culture; effective instruction; curriculum; assessment and intervention systems; effective staffing practices; enabling the effective use of data, effective use of time, and effective family and community engagement. Other considerations are job-embedded coaches, use of additional time, alignment of curriculum with standards, school safety protocols, and family and community engagement.

Using Systems: Develop a Process as Opposed to Buying a Product

Another focus of the turnaround was the establishment of "systems" so practices are embedded and not "add-ons." When we look at the Turnaround Principles we see instruction, use of data, assessments, and interventions as critical to the turnaround process, and they are all tied to the "planning stage."

The effects of Edmonds's research on Correlates of Effective Schools and the Turnaround Principles for School Improvement were very clear. The road map for correlates includes strong leadership, focus on effective instruction tied to standards-based curriculum, positive school environment, and high expectations for all students. Low-performing schools are using the current research of Turnaround Principles, which are grounded in the Effective School correlates (see the research by Blankstein 2013; Chenworth 2009; Chenworth and Theokas 2011; Reeves 2006; Reckhow 2013; Salmonowicz 2009).

Setting the Social and Emotional Environment for Learning to Occur

The social and emotional environment, as stated in the previous chapter, is a critical factor for learning. Once the emotional climate is established and the teacher plans for instructional delivery, beginning with the Readiness Set, the next logical level is the establishment of an Essential Question.

(Appendix B has a rubric that can be used to assess the classroom environment.)

On to answering the question: What is an Essential Question?

ESSENTIAL QUESTION

The Essential Question enables the student to understand the path or direction of the teacher's thinking as the long-term goal, and the objective is the short-term goal. In other words, the Essential Question is the "big idea" or concept which the objective addresses. Posting or stating an Essential Question prior to the lesson and after the Readiness Set is consistent with the brain's processing of visual information in a holistic manner.

Seeking Completeness for the Learner's Brain

In essence, the brain is looking for a pattern in what the learners see. This pattern seeking is also known as "visual thinking." Basically, the brain needs to determine whether or not there is an evident relationship to the content being taught and the big picture. The SLT (objective) answers the question what are we learning today, and the Essential Question answers the question why we are learning it. The Essential Question enables the brain to "see" the completeness. An example of the brain looking for completeness is when we are shown an optical illusion. The eyes search for a pattern, but the illusion causes the visual impression to be compromised.

Posting the Essential Question

When writing an Essential Question, one should keep in mind that it should be posted on the board for students to see. It should be placed near the SLT (objective) so the student will know what the short-term goal (SLT) and the long-term goal (Essential Question) of the lesson are.

The Essential Question and Pattern Seeking

Another way to understand the Essential Question is to see it as a relationship between the cognitive process of the new stimuli (the lesson) and the student's current frame of reference. This cognitive process is the brain's function, by which it sorts and orders new information. The learner's brain is contemplating and thinking: What is the relationship, and what is the pattern?

Patterning refers to the cognitive process of categorizing new stimuli into concepts that are alike, familiar, or novel and then combining the concepts to create new patterns of thinking and understanding. Being able to visualize and understand a relationship is a necessary skill for students in order to build sense and meaning into the lesson.

The Essential Question serves to help the student understand the relationship between the daily objective (what is being taught) and the broader, deeper concepts that the Essential Question seeks to answer. If we use the analogy of traveling on a journey, the journey would begin with a starting point, namely the SLT (objective). The DSL would be the end point or the completion of the objective. The Essential Question is the identification of the journey. The Essential Question would be "Where are we are going on our trip?"

Please refer to the rubrics at the end of the chapter that has a set of rules for writing an SLT (objective) and DSL.

The Essential Question and Self-Regulation

A posted Essential Question also helps the student begin the process of self-regulation. Self-regulation describes a process of taking control of and evaluating one's own learning and behavior. In order to take control of one's learning, the student must know what the big concept is and what is expected to frame the learning experience.

Pintrich and his colleagues (Pintrich 2004; Pintrich and DeGroot 1990; Pintrich and Zusko 2000; Pintrich, Wolter, and Baxter 2000; Wolters 2003; Wolters et. al., 2005) promote a model of self-regulated learning, which encompasses four interdependent phases. Setting goals, a core feature of all models proposed for self-regulated learning, is one key central process within this phase as well as the beginning of the self-regulation process.

Once the goals have been established, they need to be transmitted to the learner. The transmission of the goals to the learner is called the "forethought" stage. At some point in the process, it is highly probable that the teacher will involve the student in the goals-setting process; however, the teacher is usually the person who plans daily lesson and determines what students will be learning.

Goal Setting, Self-Regulation, and the Essential Question

Goal setting for the student begins when the teacher posts the Essential Question and Student Learning Target (objective) on the classroom whiteboard. It is necessary for the students to see both the Essential Question and the objective in a permanent location.

The importance of this routine posting is to build a pattern so the student can begin self-regulation immediately. In some schools, all teachers post the Essential Question and SLT in the same location so all students, no matter what class or grade level they are in, will know where to look when they enter a classroom.

Initially, the teacher's responsibility is to prompt the student to look and read the Essential Question and the SLT objective of the day. Posting the Essential Question encourages the self-regulation process, but initially it needs to be underscored by the teacher, in order to attain the desired result from the learner.

To Post or Not to Post . . . That Is the Question

Just posting an Essential Question or SLT will not get achievement results. It is unrealistic to think that just posting an Essential Question and SLT, student achievement will improve. Too often teachers are directed to post Essential Questions and SLTs. The posting is an act of compliance, but it has no value since it does not promote self-regulation.

If the teacher sees the value of the SLT and Essential Questions, he or she will refer back to the SLT (objective) using prompts or gestures. The teacher may say, "Don't forget we are learning," and then may turn and point to the objective. Teacher then helps to tie in what they are learning by reminding students throughout the lesson; "Don't forget, we are learning x, and you will show me that you mastered the skill by x."

For students in the lower grades, teachers can write "I can" statements for the objective. For the DSL, the teacher can write DSL or write: I know I have it when . . . " or the teacher can write "Show Me," which means that the student feels they know the information they show the teacher.

From Compliance to Purpose

Teachers need to move from the compliance mode to "purpose." Just like posting the Student Learning Target (SLT) and EQ for compliance has no value, the same holds true for posting rubrics or exemplars. They serve a specific purpose.

The purpose is to empower and teach the learner to be self-dependent. The learner can use the classroom environment for promoting self-regulation and self-responsibility to manage and monitor their learning. Students will not have to wait in line by the teacher's desk to be told what to do but can use the classroom environment to self-manage and self-monitor their learning. The learning environment now becomes a classroom aide or an additional teaching tool.

Stage One: The Planning Stage

The Learner's Brain Model, as described in this book, has four stages. The first stage is the planning stage.

Even though the teacher will acknowledge the Essential Question and SLT, teachers often ask the question; "Why do students forget everything I say? It seems that students can remember everything that's on television and forget everything I say?" Does that sound familiar? Often teachers wonder why students will remember songs, videos, or TV shows, but forget what is taught from the previous day.

The answer to the question is that your memory is not a product of what you want to remember. How often do teachers hear students say they studied long and hard for a test and upset when they did not get the grade they thought they should have received or got answers marked wrong which they thought they had the correct answer.

Memory is a product of what you think about. Teachers want their student to think about the information they are learning and to internalize it. As a teacher friend told me, if the student is not dreaming about algebra (the subject she taught), then he or she is not learning it.

Moving from Short-Term to Long-Term Memory

As teachers, we intuitively understand that asking students to record information or take notes during a lesson, which may be on a test or quiz, is actually focusing the student's attention to the task at hand. Since long-term learning requires moving information from short-term or working memory to long-term memory, two activities must now occur: (1) information must have meaning and make sense and (2) information must be repeated and used.

The process of retention and retrieval involves the establishment of patterns or relationships. The process of retention is aided by scaffolding or "cascading" the information. As information is presented, neural networks make the connections, so as more and more connections are made, the connections are strengthened and the action is expedited.

Eventually the message is a learned skill and becomes "procedural" or second nature as it is stored in long-term memory. Anyone who has played an instrument will know that they practice slowly to go fast. Practicing slowly helps to make neural connections. As the practice continues, the connections become second nature (muscle memory develops) and the musician is able to play faster.

For teachers the implication is to reinforce the learning using practice, application, or home learning to reinforce the skills learned. The key to remember is that practice does not make perfect. If one practices the multiplication tables incorrectly, the incorrect practice will become permanent. Perfect practice makes perfect. More importantly, teachers want their students to learn the information correctly or else teachers will have to unmake the information students learned incorrectly.

Pattern Seeking

The Learner's Brain Model involves scaffolding information during the instructional delivery. Learners are able to activate prior knowledge so that new experiences can be built into the existing patterns and relationships can be programmed.

The building of these patterns develops a connected, strengthened neural network. More importantly, the connections are similar to a holograph, whereas, when one item is retrieved, the entire connection is retrieved.

The concept of pattern seeking has implications for teachers as connections that are used are reinforced. Teachers can reinforce the learning by using practical application of skills taught or using home learning to reinforce the skills taught. As the neurons make connections and the connections are used, the connections become faster. For example, think about learning a new skill or practicing a new skill. At first one moves slowly and as he or she becomes more proficient, speed is achieved. At some point the information is in long-term memory, thus accounting for the speed. Once the information is in long-term memory, it will stay there.

Another example of pattern seeking leading to meaning is if someone who has been a plumber and is at the early stages of Alzheimer's disease, we know that the person may have difficulty in remembering things. But if he or she hears a leaky faucet, he or she will be able to fix it since the knowledge to fix it is in long-term memory. We don't actually forget things but instead we have a hard time retrieving them.

The Concept of Relevancy

A key element to establish long-term memory is to ensure that new lessons are relevant and meaningful to the student. Relevance is an important factor for students. It allows them insight into the value of what is being learned and how it can be applied to real world. It is the concept of relevance that connects sense and meaning for the student. Sense and meaning appear to be among the major criteria that the brain uses when deciding what to encode in long-term memory.

Additionally, when information makes sense, it aids in the creation and establishment of an emotional environment that is conducive to learning. When a student finds the information puzzling or when he or she cannot make sense of the subject matter, the student will intuitively ask: "why are we learning this material, or how will I use this information, or what's the point to the lesson?" These statements are not useful when establishing an emotional environment conducive for learning.

Using the Emotional Environment to Support
Sense and Meaning

A positive emotional environment supports learning. In particular, social and affective neuroscientists clearly link the interdependence of cognitive learning and the emotional environment. The importance of a positive emotional environment precedes successful learning.

The teacher plays a critical role in managing the classroom's social environment, so that optimal emotional and cognitive learning can take place and the critical factor is the preplanning which is required. When planning lessons, teachers should keep the following in mind:

- Learning is emotional; a safe emotional environment is necessary.
- Emotions are expressed verbally and visually. Sometimes our body language speaks louder than our verbal message.
- Emotions can affect future learning.
- Students will never forget how you made them feel. In some cases, that may be the only thing they remember about their teacher.

SELF-REGULATION

Self-regulation involves metacognition or thinking about one's thinking. This is an extremely important concept of the learning process as it develops self-regulated learners. Learners who are able to self-monitor, self-manage, or self-learn will be more successful in their academic careers. As scholars become twenty-first-century learners, they need to have the capacity to know how to regulate and monitor their time and themselves during this time.

Promoting Strategies for Self-Regulation

The process of self-regulation is demonstrated in a variety of ways. One way is for the teacher to model the process in the classroom. The process must be taught, so the student will know what strategies to employ for self-regulation. For example, when students engage in note-taking, the teacher instructs the students to refer back to their notes, and observe the relationship between the short- and long-term goals in the presented material.

In order to evoke self-regulation strategies, the teacher will tell the students to write the SLT (objective) on the top of their note page, so when it's time to review the notes, the students will see the relationship of their notes to the specific SLT (objective). The students can also seek out other resources and information to address the specific SLT (objective).

The seeking out of information and the development of metacognition skills are consistent with Self Regulation Learning (SRL). These types of activities begin the process of developing a "habit of mind" and/or disposition to self-motivate, thereby coming full circle and continually seeking out more or new information. This will develop an intrinsic "want" within the student for learning.

In order to stress student ownership, the writer encourages teachers to use "I" when writing the SLT (objective). The use of "I" helps personalize the learning, promote students' self-identity, and direct self-regulation.

For information about writing objectives and DSLs, a rubric that has "indicators" listed is available to use for self-assessment.

Promoting Self-Regulation Strategies

Self-regulation strategies and metacognition do have an impact on student learning and achievement at all levels. As Self-Regulation strategies must be learned, teachers should begin the process as soon as possible. In order for the teacher to teach self regulation skills, it requires having the student's attention. Student attention is also necessary for initiating memory.

Teachers can prompt the student's attention by using reminders such as "today we are focusing on x, and don't forget x." The teacher should point to the objective and Essential Question and instruct the students to do a peer share about what they are learning today. During the lesson the teacher should focus the student's attention by using gestures, prompts, and explanations regarding how the new material correlates to the long- and short-term goals.

The prompting process can be done at critical times throughout the lesson. By focusing the students' attention strategically, the teacher will encourage the students to begin constructing meaning ideas for themselves about the subject matter.

Creating Mindfulness

Mindfulness, or creating the most effective student frame of mind and thinking, is essential when teachers use prompting. The teacher should defer to the SLT (objective) and be cognizant of strategic prompting or else the lesson will backfire and eventually turn the student away from making the needed meaningful connections to the lesson. Timing is crucial, and an inert teacher's ability to understand his or her audience is an integral part of delivering this method properly.

Making Memory

Teachers should also be mindful that memory is a by-product of what the student is thinking. Memory is also promoted by strategies that engender an analysis of the material, encouraging students to compare and contrast what they are learning.

It is important for teachers to help regulate and access students' working memory to begin the brain's processing and thinking about the task. To determine memory, researchers were able to see what part of the brain was engaged using fMRIs when a person is told something, when he or she hears something, when he or she says something, or when he or she thinks about something. A greater area of the brain is engaged when one thinks about something in contrast to when one states it.

Selective Focus

When we begin to understand the importance of selective attention, we may ask ourselves about the implications for selective focus, especially when doing word problems. When students are faced with word problems, they must read the problem and decide what information is relevant and what information is a detractor. The "relevant" information must be retained, and the irrelevant information must be dismissed.

For example, if one was given a word problem such as what is the day after the day after tomorrow, if the day before the day before yesterday is Monday? Let's remember that the question to address first in this word problem is what information is valuable and important and what information is a distraction.

The only real information that we are able to determine is that the day before the day before yesterday is Monday. So we start our problem with this relevant information. We think the day before, day before yesterday is Monday then:

Table 2.1.   Possible Solution to Math problem

DBDBY	DBY	Yesterday	Today	Tomorrow	DAT	DADAT
Monday	Tuesday	Wednesday	Thursday	Friday	Saturday	Sunday

The problem is also solved mathematically. When thinking about the day before the day before yesterday is Monday, we designate it as an "x." The day before yesterday would be subtracting a day, but you are NOT starting at Monday, you are starting at an unknown day. So you have to work backward, instead of subtracting 1, you have to add 1 for each day.

Therefore, $x + 1 + 1 + 1$ would be the equation for the day before the day before yesterday (because yesterday is +1, the day before yesterday is +1, and the day before the day is + 1). Combine like terms and the equation is $x + 3$, which is Monday plus 3 days and that = Thursday.

For the next part we say, the day after the day after tomorrow and we think, we are now starting with Thursday. Since you know the start date you do NOT have to work backward from here.

Next, make Thursday = y

Therefore, $y + 1 + 1 + 1$ would be the equation for the day after the day after tomorrow (because tomorrow is +1, the day after tomorrow is +1, and the day after the day is +1). Combine like terms and the equation is $y + 3$, which is Thursday plus 3 days = Sunday. That is your answer!

It is apparent that word problems are very demanding on our working memory and our working memory is affected by selected attention.

WRITING THE SLT (OBJECTIVE)

In the preplanning stage, teachers should keep in mind the "big picture" or major standards to be learned. Keeping the desired result in mind will enable a teacher to focus on the types of questions that will be used in the lesson to achieve the desired result. This is an important aspect of lesson design.

As teacher questions are developed, they will be useful in guiding the student's discovery. Additionally, the level of difficulty for the activity can be used to promote higher-level thinking. Keeping the end in mind will enable a teacher to preplan the kinds and types of questioning data that will be used in the lesson, the level of difficulty which will be addressed, and a variety of questions which will be determined about how the student will comprehend all of the skills being presented. These questions should and could promote student curiosity.

Students Are Naturally Curious but Not Necessarily Good Thinkers Unless . . .

When planning the lesson, teachers should tap upon students' natural curiosity. Although students are naturally curious, they may not be good thinkers, unless the teacher sets the conditions for cognitive inquiry. Absent of cognitive stimulation, students will fail to see the importance of what they are learning or, more importantly, they will not be cognitively challenged.

Every teacher knows the effect of challenging students or adding some degree of a challenge to the learner. This poses the question in the minds of teachers and other thinkers: "How do we get students to start thinking?"

Two necessary components for learning are making sense and having meaning. We should remember that in order for information to move from short- to long-term memory, developing sense and having meaning is a necessary precondition for long-term memory.

Information that has survival value will get immediate attention and will be quickly stored into long-term memory. As well as survival meaning, emotional experience, both good and bad, will also get stored. Who among us can't remember a good or bad emotional experience? After the readiness activity, the teacher begins the process of "making" sense and developing meaning from the material.

How Is Making Sense and Promoting Meaning Developed by the Teacher?

The teacher starts the process by pointing the student in the right direction. As noted, the SLT (objectives) are posted and the students begin to identify with and/or articulate them. This sequence begins with the "pointing in the right direction" process. Therefore, a safe and secure environment, in addition to posted SLT (objectives) that are "student friendly," ensures that the students will learn what is expected of them from each individual lesson.

With compliance and regulations in mind, teachers often post detailed SLT (objectives) that are geared to administrative requirement and with less thought in mind for the students. The teacher may inadvertently fail to see the value of posting SLT (objectives) and how it should be used for students' self-regulation.

An SLT (objective) posted for an administrator so that the teacher can rid himself or herself of the many requirements and demands placed upon him or her in the classroom is the ultimate compliant mind-set. Ultimately, this mind-set will only lead to deeper and larger teaching issues.

Killer Question: Will This Be on the Test?

Teachers will quickly know if the student is not engaged in the lesson or does not understand the lesson objective when a student asks: Will this be on the test? What he or she is saying is that this information has no meaning to him or her. There is little or no relationship between the SLT (objective) and what the student needs to know. The student may think that the information is not useful. If, however, it is going to be on a test, then the student thinks that paying attention is warranted to some degree.

This was apparent to the author when he taught undergraduate students at the university level. During an instructional period where direct instruction was being used, a student asked: Is this going to be on the test? The reply was that the information was background information and was not going to be on the test. Almost immediately, everyone put their pencils down and stopped taking notes. This was quite a "wake-up" call.

The information made sense to the students but did not have meaning or significance to them. Therefore, they felt that it was not necessary to pay 100 percent attention to the direct instruction. When the experience was relayed to a university colleague, she replied, "Tell the students that the information *could* be on the test." This sounded like good advice.

A Lesson Learned

During the following class, the hope was that the same student would repeat history and ask me if any of the information being taught would be on the test. Perhaps the student figured he could streamline his note-taking this way and my answer would determine what he would write.

When he asked this time, the reply was, "Yes, this information could very well show up on your test." Because of the response, the student who asked the question and the other undergraduate students in the room continued to take notes.

When viewing the diligent note-taking, it was obvious for the need to distinguish between important information and the so-called background information or the students would be scripting during the whole lesson, participating less, and would not gain as much sense and meaning from the lesson.

Telling the students what information would be used at a later date helped them understand and develop better note-taking skills so eventually they would be determining what information was important. If students are constantly script-taking, they will miss the discussion during the lesson.

Teachers who have students read a paragraph out loud in class quickly realize that when they ask the student what did the paragraph say, the normal student response is: "I don't know." The reason they are not aware of what the paragraph said is that they focused on each word they were reading and not the meaning of what they were reading.

Questions Which Indicate That Students Do Not See the Value in What Is Being Taught

The "Is this going to be on the test today" question is indicative of the students not finding value in what is being taught. Another question that is an indication that the process is lacking sense and meaning is when the student says, "Do we have to know this?" Again the answer is the same. The students are expressing in no uncertain terms that the information has no meaning to them unless it's going to be tested or on a quiz sometime in their near future.

Students may be able to remember information in a twenty-four-hour time period, but lack the ability to retain it for longer period of time. Of course, there may be times when a student is attempting to seek understanding and meaning from the lesson, so he or she will need clarification and will ask, "Why do we have to know this?"

In this particular venue, the student is really striving to make sense of the information presented to him or her. The teacher may find that the student may seem puzzled and a lack of understanding of the lesson in a statement such as, "This doesn't make sense." What the student is conveying is that he or she fails to see the value of lesson information and since the lesson's SLT (objective) was not clear to him or her from the onset, there was little or no sense and meaning developed throughout the lesson.

The Resolution to Killer Questions

The resolution to the previous types of questions is simple: the information must be relevant, meaningful, and linked to the student's frame of reference, so that the student can activate prior knowledge to help interpret this new information.

During the beginning of a lesson, a teacher is aware of what he or she expects from the students during the lesson. While that teacher is proceeding with the lesson, he or she is also informally evaluating the progress of the students' understanding of the delivered material.

A master teacher will want to spark the student interest as he or she teaches to keep the students actively listening and engaged. He or she will plan and implement precise questioning as the lesson proceeds. These questions will act as prompts or motivators to activate student interest.

Making Predictions

An excellent way to get students to be attentive and spark their interest is to have them make predictions. Neuroscientists know and appreciate the value of prediction. Predictions increase attention and memory as the predictors will be eager to know if their prediction was accurate. Solving a problem is not only is exciting, but when one solves a problem the brain rewards itself with a neurotransmitter called dopamine. That neurotransmitter stimulates the brain's pleasure system. Once students are making predictions and they are correct, the neurotransmitter is emitted.

Predictions can be extremely useful in getting students interested in the lesson. We have seen students wait with baited breath, to see if their prediction was correct! If they were correct we see high fives, air pumps, or smiles. The teacher can build on his or her questioning by stating, "What do you think will happen next?" This type of questioning, during strategic times in the instruction, will help to promote the students' thinking. It's notable that pleasure comes from solving the problem.

Students who are making limited progress, while working on solutions, will not enjoy the activity, and therefore the result will not be a pleasurable feeling for such students. Even if the content of a problem may be sufficient to prompt students' interest at first, it will not maintain attention for a long period of time, hence the need to prompt interest through prediction.

PREDICTION

The process of prediction begins with the construction of the SLT (objective). When developing your SLT (objective), the teacher should think of questions which will encourage the students to predict what will happen before they begin work on their problems.

As teachers work on the SLT (objective), it is important to begin to direct their thoughts to probing questions to promote prediction. The purpose of pre-developing questions, prior to the lesson, is that the teacher will have a number of questions to use during the course of the lesson. The questions will focus the students' thoughts on their prediction.

Teachers may not feel having predetermined questions is useful as they feel they can develop questions during the "flow" of the class. This thinking leaves the process up to chance. Although teachers may be able to think of probing questions during the lesson, it is better to have the questions preplanned.

Preplanning questions are also necessary when the teachers know that there may be a place in the lesson where students will be stuck. What questions can be asked to help redirect student thinking since the teacher recognizes that it will occur in certain parts of the lesson?

Plan questions that scaffold up to help the student reach a deeper level of thinking. Plan questions that formulate questions that puzzle the students and to make them curious. The puzzlement and inquisitiveness will help the students focus on deciphering information and determining what will be necessary to resolve the problem.

Unless the cognitive conditions are conducive for learning and students are challenged, students will avoid thinking and prefer to be told what to do. How often has a teacher been asked what do you want? Or, a teacher's sample model is provided and the final student product looks exactly like the teacher model.

Preplanning the Lesson

In the preplanning stage, every teacher must address how to teach students to be critical thinkers and problem solvers so they can do their own creative, independent work and not replicate a teacher's model.

Preplanning is also important as time is the teacher's enemy, so "well begun is half done." Teachers must meet deadlines and ready their students for high-stake standardized testing. Pressure to get in all the information necessary to pass the high-stakes tests often affects the pace of the lesson and the lesson becomes accelerated.

The reality is that teachers must teach facts and information that will appear on the high-stake tests. All persons involved in education recognize that high-stakes testing is a practical reality and soon will be used for assessing teacher effectiveness if not done already in some states. The question of high-stakes testing will be addressed more fully during the chapter 4 on Input.

The answer regarding high-stake testing is that research from cognitive science has shown that the skills that teachers want students to master, such as the ability to analyze and think critically, require students to build on their factual base by applying what they know. The adage is: If you teach for competency (skills and facts), you may not get performance (application); if you teach for performance, you automatically get competency (since you need facts and skills to be able to apply them via application).

Research on Goal Setting

The research about goal setting and/or objectives is very clear. Marzano, Pickering, and Pollock, in their work, *Classroom Instruction That Works* (2001), identify seeking objectives and providing feedback as a critical component for student success. In their text, they cite three studies that articulate the value of objectives. Specifically, Wise and Okey (1983) studied the general effect on setting objectives and observed the impact they had on student success. They discovered that setting objectives and goals yielded percentage gains of 41 percentage points in three studies and 18 percentage points in twenty-five studies.

Walberg (1999) also focused on the general effect of setting goals or objectives, and the gain was 18 percent improvement in the twenty-one studies that were reviewed. Finally, an analysis of 204 studies conducted by Lipsey and Wilson (1993) revealed a percentage gain of 21 points. (Marzano, Pickering, and Pollock 2001, 93). Clearly, this research verifies that setting objectives (short term) and goals (long term) provide positive results relative to student achievement.

How Is an Objective Developed?

The SLT (objective) has two components: the condition, which is the teacher's delivery system (i.e., lecture, small group), and behavior, which is what the student will be learning. There is a companion component to the objective and that is how the learning will be measured, which is the Demonstration of Student Learning (DSL).

The two components are like bookends as the SLT (objective) starts the process of teacher instruction to the learner and the DSL is the measurement of the learning. In between the two bookends is the instructional delivery and student self-regulation. For students, the teacher can write a student-friendly SLT (objective) of what the students will be learning and a DSL that informs the students on how they will be assessed.

For administrators, there is also another part called "condition," which is the instructional strategy that a teacher will use to deliver the lesson. It is important to note that the condition part of the SLT objective is valuable for an administrator. The administrator will see the instructional strategies a teacher plans to use and has used over the course of the year.

Writing the Student Learning Target (Objective)

When writing a SLT objective, the task is to focus on the student and not on developing a SLT objective written for the administrator. The teacher should ask: What do I expect the student to know and do and how will I know that the student has learned it? If those questions are to be considered, the teacher will write the SLT: "I will be able to do. . . ." Once that aspect of the SLT objective is developed, the teacher will be able to determine how students will demonstrate their knowledge.

The Demonstration of Student Learning (DSL) can be written: I will be able to demonstrate, explain, justify, show, or other higher-level verbs that promote metacognition. When writing the SLT (objective) and DSL, there are questions the teachers can ask themselves.

Questions to Ask When Considering Behavior

What do I want my students to learn? How will I use questioning to promote the desired behavior? How will I know students are learning the material?

These questions develop immediate clarification for the teacher and helps him or her to order his or her thinking skills with his or her lesson design. After establishing that the teacher can focus on his or her questioning techniques, his or her objective, and his or her goals, then and only then will the behavior question lead to the part of the objective which is "condition."

Questions to Ask When Considering "Condition"

Have I used a varied approach in my instructional delivery? (This is important for the administrator and not the student, as the student will not have control over how the teacher presents the lesson). What instruction method or framework am I going to provide to the student to address the learning question?

The condition question begins a thought process regarding what the teacher had ordered in his or her mind from the onset of the lesson. It provides the teacher a sequencing technique for starting a lesson. It also ensures that the student has learned the objectives of the lesson. The teacher then evaluates his or her lesson by deciding whether the students are addressing the instructional question. He or she would do this by assessment, both formal and informal.

Questions to Ask When Considering Assessment

How will the students demonstrate mastery of the skills presented? How will I help the students to regulate their own learning? What are multiple pathways I can use for the students to show mastery?

Mastery of the lesson will be demonstrated by a DSL. When mastery is achieved, the student will be able to easily retrieve this information from long-term memory and apply it to new learning. The teacher will be able to observe this application of information through any means of assessments.

DOMAINS OF LEARNING FOR THE STUDENT LEARNING TARGET (OBJECTIVE)

When constructing an SLT (objective), teachers should be mindful of the cognitive, affective, psychomotor, and metacognitive levels of student thinking.

The cognitive domain addresses the knowledge, thinking stage. What is it that the teacher wants the student to learn?

The affective domain addresses feeling and attitudes. How will the student be synthesizing information, reacting to comments, organizing and conceptualizing information, reflecting on information, and expressing their opinion?

The psychomotor domain addresses doing, constructing, designing, demonstrating, manipulating, articulating, performing, and other action verbs. This domain can also be the measurement (DSL) of the learning target.

The verbs that are used in the SLT (objectives) will have an impact on the kinds of activities used in the lesson. At an initial workshop on writing STLs objectives and DSLs, this notion was tested. At the conclusion of the initial workshop, a follow-up activity occurred whereby the teachers came to the workshop with objectives and DSLs they had written.

A rubric was used (refer to appendix A for rubric) to evaluate the SLT objective relative to the verbs used. After teachers evaluated the SLT objective using the rubric, they changed the verbs in the SLT objective as a test to see what would happen. It was amazing to see how the discussion changed! With the new verbs, which were at a higher level on Revised Bloom's Taxonomy (RBT), the activities changed.

A conversation focused on the types of verbs used, and it promoted what kinds of student actions are planned. Teachers began to discuss changes they needed to make if they wanted creativity from their students. The teachers were amazed that changing verbs caused the student engagement activities to change.

All the discussion about using higher-level verbs was not as effective as having teachers actually doing an activity in which they would take an objective and change the verbs in it. Teachers had learned a highly valuable lesson. The supervisor and principal could not have been more pleased with the results and the revelations that were discovered in the room on that day.

How the SLT objective will be addressed is the next consideration.

WRITING THE DSL

Important considerations are as follows:

- The DSL should tie directly into the lesson SLT objective and the guaranteed curriculum and should not be a stand-alone activity but a measurement of what was taught. Remember, the DSL measures what was taught.
- The DSL can usually be accomplished in a short period of time and will not require more than ten minutes. Use the DSL after each lesson, so if two different lessons were taught in an eighty-minute block to time, there will be two DSLs planned.
- The use of higher-level verbs in the DSL will promote metacognition.
- The DSL varies according to what was taught and can be expressed using "multiple pathways."
- The DSL can be developed based on the student's multiple intelligences (i.e., verbal linguistic students can do a written task; mathematical students can incorporate an equation or puzzle) and can be performance-based.

Student-Friendly DSLs

Another important aspect of writing the DSL is to make it "student-friendly." The purpose of this is so the student will be able to articulate what he or she is expected to learn. This is directly related to why the model stresses using "I" instead of Student Will Be Able to or Learner Will Be Able to or We Are Learning Today when writing objectives. The use of "I" for the SLT objective and the DSL will promote four important considerations for the student:

- Self-motivation—This is what I am learning and how I will be assessed so I need to pay attention in class as I am going to be assessed on what is being taught.
- Self-regulation—How will I monitor and regulate my learning throughout the lesson? What rubrics do I need to be successful?
- Self-efficacy—How will I internalize the information?
- Self-assessments—How will I monitor my learning or assess my understanding throughout the lesson? Enter the Readiness Set.

READINESS SET

The purpose of the Readiness Set is to focus student attention. Just telling students to focus will not work. An example is an activity conducted in one of my graduate classes.

The activity was the man in a gorilla suit video. It involves watching a video in which the viewer counts the number of basketball passes a team of three people passed. The activity involved three students wearing white shirts and three students wearing black shirts. Students were asked to count the number of passes made by students wearing black shirts. In essence, students were to focus their attention on the black-shirted players and their passing of the ball.

The prompt to only watch one group of students serves to draw attention to only the students with black shirts. During the course of the passing, a student dressed in a gorilla suit walked into the middle of the gymnasium, through the students passing the ball, stops, and beat his chest. The "gorilla" then proceeds to walk out of the gymnasium.

What is amazing is that at the end of the video, when asked how many passes were thrown, most folks would answer either 17 or 18.

Did You See the Gorilla?

When asked did they see the person in a gorilla suit? Students were in disbelief! Yes, about halfway through the basketball passing activity, a person dressed in a gorilla suit walks through the students passing the ball, beats his chest, and continues walking out of sight. About 50 percent of the class said that they saw it happen, while the other half sat in disbelief. When the video was replayed, the 50 percent of students who did not see the person in the gorilla suit were then able to point him out the second time. Needless to say, this 50 percent of students, who were teachers, were quite embarrassed that they missed it in the first place!

Initially, the class was directed to focus their attention on counting passes and nothing else, so other information was blocked out. This activity was courtesy of Surprising Studies of Visual Awareness, VisCog Productions. This was a wonderful example of focused attention. So, to reiterate, focusing the student's attention to the players in the basketball activity equates to having the objective on the board and focusing the student attention.

Focusing Student Attention

One way to focus attention is after the Readiness Set is introduced; ask the students to look at the SLT objective on the board (objective verification). A comment from the teacher like "today's lesson is tied to the posted SLT objective" will provide objective verification and help the student "contextualize" the learning.

Is This Going to Be on the Test?

We are aware of this question when we are teaching a lesson. As noted in prior pages of this text, this professor has determined that the answer of YES is always applicable. Having students do objective verification will help them frame the lesson and contextualize what they are learning. The focus is on learning and not the test.

Objective Verification and Vision Processing

Encouraging students to refocus on the objective after the Readiness Set is important because vision is an important function, which doesn't require thought. We take in information through our senses, and it is processed in our short-term memory. As such, the brain filters the information to determine if it is valuable.

Information that does not have value is discarded, as opposed to information that makes sense and has meaning. By refocusing the student back to the objective, it helps the brain to pay attention and process information that will now have sense and meaning.

Another way to promote "value" or at least focus is to use color.

- Color may be used to give clues to the brain, about where to locate information or an object in the classroom.
- The careful use of bold colors, such as red or orange, will provoke student interest.
- The international ranking of colors to demand attention is blue, red, green, violet, orange, and lemony yellow.
- An occasional bold stroke of red or orange attracts the learner's attention to detail.
- Both red and orange are used for alerting children to specific points of knowledge or new concepts.

Keeping this research regarding colors in mind, teachers should be mindful of colors that they present in the classroom and also their choices of colors for writing objectives on the board.

SETTING THE CLASSROOM ENVIRONMENT

What becomes critical is for the teacher to understand how significantly important a person's emotions are in the educational process. Recognizing the value of emotions and by providing a safe environment for the student, teachers can encourage students to establish classroom rules. By empowering students to become part of the process of establishing rules, the end result will be that the student will support the consequences. There is more student buy-in when they develop their rules. A win-win situation.

Another consideration for teachers is to know that students are in touch with their emotions, since emotions are an unconscious arousal system and education is emotional.

By providing a safe and orderly school environment, as well as encouraging students to be cognizant of stress reduction, conflict management, and biofeedback, a safe emotional environment is established.

Twenty-First-Century Learning in a Safe Classroom Environment

How then has safe environment research been applied to the classroom? The new view of learning draws upon various research done in cognitive neuroscience, cognitive psychology, brain research, and artificial intelligence.

The new view of twenty-first-century learning is expressed simply in terms of the following:

- Students are the learners and must construct understanding for themselves.
- Information is important but understanding and applying concepts, relationships, and patterns activate deeper and longer-lasting learning.
- Knowing relationships depends on having prior knowledge.
- The use of visuals and applying information promotes retention.

Learning is more than teachers lecturing and students sitting at their desks taking notes. A more effective process is for learners to be involved in the learning activity and interact with their environment. This implies that a student must feel safe in the classroom environment and feel free to try and even make mistakes.

Taking in Information Using More Than One Modality

Using multiple senses to process information is important as learners store components and images in various places. Items that are similar are stored together.

For example, there is storage space for shapes, color, movement, sequence, and textures. The brain makes interwoven connections and stores items in clusters. The critical factor is the quality of the connection and how well the brain organizes and stores the relationships between (and among) the various events and aspects.

Prior knowledge is used to interpret new material and wherever bits of information are isolated from these systems are forgotten and they become inaccessible to memory. They become orphans and will not stay in memory long. One way to activate prior knowledge is to encourage students to explore, touch, manipulate, and test theories because that helps to reconstruct the student's learning and brings meaning to this learning.

Did You BK Today?

The symbol is linked to an image.

Rehearsal Teaching

The new curriculum approach of linking the old with the new includes using concepts like "rehearsal teaching." The concept involves reinforcing what has been learned. The rehearsal provides knowledge construction and reinforcement thereby making the concept permanent. The next step is to add something new to the equation so the brain can use the prior knowledge to assimilate the new knowledge, thereby making a connection of the old with the new.

Rehearsal Teaching versus Practice

This notion of rehearsal is different from practice. Practice is repetition of a task to improve the performance of the task. When playing an instrument, the musician will practice scales to improve his or her performance. The practice will involve slowing and correctly playing the scale. The concept for developing speed and proficiency for scales is to "practice slowly to get fast." In essence, slow and methodical practice will reinforce proper position and develop muscle memory. Eventually, the practice speed will be increased to the desired level.

Rehearsal, on the other hand, endeavors to promote learning, by allowing the brain to recognize that the task that is being learned is not task-specific but transferable and can be used in a variety of ways, other than only in one particular way. The rehearsals will strengthen the connections among and between the various storage areas. A critical factor is to establish the environment to allow for rehearsals and to promote student self-regulation.

Reflective questions for a teacher to ask for integrating new knowledge in a well-established environment:

- How will I establish the classroom environment to encourage student autonomy, interaction, and leadership?
- Is the SLT objective achievable in one class period?
- What verbs will I use to promote cognition?
- How will students demonstrate that they know the skills which were taught? Will I plan frequent checks for understanding so I can monitor and adjust the lesson?
- Will I refer back to the SLT via prompts or gestures to help students develop sense and meaning throughout the lesson?
- What data do I need to collect during and after the lesson to plan subsequent lessons?
- What DSL am I going to plan to measure what was taught?
- Am I going to use higher-level verbs to remote metacognition?
- Will the assessments be rigorous?
- Did I plan what questions I am going to ask throughout the lesson?
- Do I know where in the lesson students will have difficulty? What do I have planned when students reach the point where there is difficulty?

The concept of teaching becomes more than the old stand-and-deliver model. The teachers will have to construct activities and experiences in an interactive environment. Teachers will have to develop lessons that promote rigor and student self-regulation. The lesson planning involves the following:

- Establishing a safe emotional environment that considers how rules will be established; will restorative practices be implemented?
- Am I planning a behavioral support program for students experiencing problems?
- How will I establish student self-regulation? Will I do it by promoting the use of rubrics, exemplars, and anchor charts?
- What questions and procedures will I use to promote student self-regulation?
- Am I planning "productive struggle" in the lesson?
- Is gradual release planned?
- Am I planning a multisensory approach in the lesson?
- Did I plan closure?
- Am I going to exit tickets?
- How will I triangular all the data for future lessons?

The next chapter will move from the planning stage to lesson delivery.

BIBLIOGRAPHY

Barbara, Z., ed. 1991. *Teaching for Intelligence*. Thousand Oaks, CA: Corwin Press.

Barnard-Brak, L., Wand Lan, and V. Paton. 2010. "Profiles and Self-Regulated Learning in the Online Learning Network: Research in Open and Distance Learning." *International Review* 1 (L): 61–73.

Blankstein, A. 2013. *Failure Is Not an Option*, 3rd edition. Thousand Oaks, CA: Corwin Press.

Bransford, John D., Ann L. Brown, and Rodney Cockings, eds. 2000. *How People Learn: Brain, Mind, Experience, and School*. Washington, DC: The National Academies Press.

Chenoweth, Karin. 2009. *How It's Being Done*. Cambridge, MA: Harvard Education Press.

Chenoweth, Karin, and C. Theokas. 2011. *Getting It Done: Leading Academic Success in Unexpected Schools*. Cambridge, MA: Harvard Education Press.

Clifford, M. M. 1984. "Thoughts on a Theory of Constructive Failure." *Educational Psychologist* 19: 108–20.

Cooper, G., and J. Sweller. 1987. "The Effect of Schema Acquisition and Rule Automation on Mathematical Problem-Solving Transfer." *Journal of Educational Psychology* 79: 347–62.

Ebbinghaus, Hermann. 1885. *Memory: A Contribution to Experimental Psychology.* Translated by Henry A. Ruger and Clara E. Bussenius, 1913 edition. New York: Teachers College.

Guttentag, Robert E. June 1989. "Age Differences in Dual-Task Performance: Procedures, Assumptions, and Results." *Developmental Review* 9 (2): 146–70.

Hardiman, M. 2010. "The Creative-Artistic Brain." In *Mind, Brain, and Education: Neuroscience Implications for the Classroom*, edited by D. Sousa, 226–46. Bloomington, IN: Solution Tree Press.

Heinich, R., M. Molenda, J. Russell, and S. Smaldino. 2002. *Instructional Media and Technologies for Learning*, 7th edition. Englewood Cliffs, NJ: Prentice Hall, Inc.

Hermans, R., and P. R. Pintrich. 2008. "Development of the Beliefs about Primary Education Scale: Distinguishing a Developmental and Transmissive Dimension." *Teaching and Teacher Education* 24 (1): 127–39.

Kirschner, P. A., J. Sweller, and R. E. Clark. 2006. "While Minimal Guidance during Instruction Does Not Work: An Analysis of the Failure of Constructivist, Discovery, Problem-Based, Experimental and Inquiry-Based Teaching." *Educational Psychologist* 41: 75–86.

Knight, Jim. 2011. *Unmistakable Impact: A Partnership Approach for Dramatically Improving Instruction.* Thousand Oaks, CA: Corwin Press.

Lipsey, M. W., and D. B. Wilson. 1993. "The Efficacy of Psychological, Educational, and Behavioral Treatment." *American Psychologist* 48 (12): 1181–1209.

Marzano, R. J. 2007. *The Art and Science of Teaching: A Comprehension Framework for Effective Instruction.* Alexandria, VA: Association for Supervision and Curriculum Development.

———. 2009. *Designing and Teaching Learning Goals and Objectives.* Alexandria, VA: Association for Supervision and Curriculum Development.

Marzano, R. J., Debra J. Pickering, and W. Pollock. 2001. *Classroom Instruction That Works.* Alexandria, VA: Association for Supervision and Curriculum Development.

Marzano, R. J., T. Waters, and B. A. McNulty. 2005. *School Leadership That Works: From Research to Results.* Alexandria, VA: Association for Supervision and Curriculum Development.

Nicol, D. J., and D. Macfarlane-Dick. 2006. "Formative Assessment and Self-Regulated Learning: A Model and Seven Principles of Good Feedback Practice." *Studies in Higher Education* 31 (2): 199–218.

O'Sullivan, J. T., and M. Pressley. 1984. "Completeness of Instruction and Strategy Transfer." *Journal of Experimental Child Psychology* 38: 275–88.

Paris, S. C., and A. H. Paris. 2001. "Classroom Applications of Research on Self-Regulate Learning." *Educational Psychologist* 36 (2): 89–101.

Pashier, H., P. Bain, B. Bottge, A. Graesser, K. Koedinger, M. McDaniel, and J. Metcalfe. 2007. *Organizing Instruction and Study to Improve Student Learning* (NCER 2007–2004). Washington, DC: National Center for Education Research, Institute of Education Sciences, US Department of Education. http://ncer.ed.gov.

Pintrich, P. R. 2000. "The Role of Goal Orientation in Self-Regulated Learning." In *Handbook of Self-Regulation*, edited by M. Boekaerts, P. R. Pintrich, and M. Zeidner, 451–502. San Diego, CA: Academic Press.

Pintrich, P. R., and E. V. De Groot. 1990. "Motivational and Self-Regulated Learning Components of Classroom Academic Performance." *Journal of Educational Psychology* 82: 33–40.

Pintrich, P. R., C. Wolters, and G. Baxter. 2000. "Assessing Metacognition and Self-Regulated Learning." In *Issues in the Measurement of Metacognition*, edited by G. Schraw and J. Impara. Lincoln, NE: Buros Institute of Mental Measurements.

Pintrich, P. R., and A. Zusho. 2002. "The Development of Academic Self-Regulation: The Role of Cognitive and Motivational Factors." In *Development of Achievement Motivation*, edited by A. Wigfield and J. S. Eccles, 249–284. Cambridge, MA: Academic Press.

Presseisen, Barbara Z., ed. 1999. *Teaching for Intelligence*. Thousand Oaks, CA: Corwin Press.

Reckhow, S. 2013. *Follow the Money: How Foundation Dollars Change Public School*. New York: Oxford University Press.

Reeves, D. R. 2004. *Accountability for Learning: How Teachers and School Leaders Can Take Change*. Alexandria, VA: Association for Supervision and Curriculum Development.

Reid, M. K., and J. G. Borkowski. 1987. "Causal Attributions of Hyperactive Children: Implications for Teaching Strategies and Self-Control." *Journal of Educational Psychology* 79 (3): 296–307.

Renkl, A. 1997. "Learning from Worked Out Examples: A Study on Individual Differences." *Cognitive Science* 21: 1–29.

Salmonowicz, M. 2009. "Meeting the Challenge of School Turnaround: Lessons from the Intersection of Research and Practice." *Phi Delta Kappan* 91 (3): 19–24.

Schunk, D. H., and J. L. Meece, eds. 1992. *Student Perceptions in the Classroom*. Hillsdale, NJ: Lawrence Erlbaum Associates Publishers.

Sousa, D., Posner, M., Willis, J., Immordine-Yang, M. H., Faeth, M., Williams, D., O'Loughlin, T., Eddu, M. D., Coch, D., Devlin, K., Dehaene, S., Ansari, D., Hardiman, M. M., Fisher, K. W., and Heikkinen, K., eds. 2010. *Mind, Brain, and Education*. Bloomington, IN: Solution Tree Press.

Sparrow, L., H. Sparrow, and P. Swan. 2000. *Student Centered Learning: Is It Possible?* In *Flexible Futures in Tertiary Teaching*, edited by A. Herrmann and M. M. Kulski. Retrieved from Proceedings of the 9th Annual Teaching Learning Forum, February 2–4, 2000, Perth: Curtin University of Technology. http://lsn.curtin.edu.au/tlf/tlf2000/sparrow.htmlman.

Sweller, J., and G. A. Cooper. 1985. "The Use of Worked Examples as a Substitute for Problem Solving in Learning Algebra." *Cognition and Instruction* 2: 59–89.

Trafton, J. A., Reiser, B. J., Keil, F., Leinhardt, G., Ram, A., Roschelle, Frank, R., Jusczyk, F. W., Mac Whinney, B., Jacobs, R., Plaut, D., Behrmann, M., Kaebling, L., Maes, P., and Presenter Vera, A. 1993. "The Contribution of Studying Examples and Solving Problems to Skill Acquisition." In M. Polson, ed. Retrieved from Proceedings of the 15th Annual Conference of the Cognitive Science Society. Hillsdale, NJ: Erlbaum Publishing.

VisCog Productions. *Surprising Studies of Visual Awareness*, Volumes 1 and 2. www.viscog.com.

Walberg, H. J. 1999. "Productive Teaching." In *New Directions for Teaching Practice and Research*, edited by H. C. Waxman and H. J. Walberg, 75–104. Berkeley, CA: McCutchen.

Wiggins, J., and J. McTighe. 2007. *Understanding by Design*. Alexandria, VA: Association for Supervision and Curriculum Development.

Willingham, D. 2010. *Why Students Don't Like School*. San Francisco, CA: Jossey-Boss.

Willis, J. May 9, 2010. *Psychology Today*. www.psychologytoday.com/blog/radical-teaching/201005/want-children-pay-attention-make-their-brains-curious.

Wise, K. C., and J. R. Okey. 1983. "A Meta-Analysis of the Effects of Various Science Teaching Strategies on Achievement." *Journal of Research in Science Teaching* 20 (5): 415–25.

Wolters, C. A. 2003. "Understanding Procrastination from a Self-Regulated Learning Perspective." *Journal of Educational Psychology* 95: 179–187.

Wolters, C. A., P. R. Pintrich, and S. A. Karabenick. 2005. "Assessing Academic Self-Regulated Learning." In *What Do Children Need to Flourish?: Conceptualizing and Measuring Indicators of Positive Development*, edited by K. A. Moore and L. H. Lippman, 251–270. New York: Springer.

Zhu, X., and H. A. Simon. 1987. "Learning/Mathematics from Examples and by Doing." *Cognition and Instruction* 4: 137–66.

Zimmerman, B. J. 1998. "Academic Studying in the Development of Personal Skill: A Self-Regulatory Perspective." *Educational Psychologist* 33 (2/3): 73–86.

———. 2009. "Theories of Self-Regulated Learning and Academic Achievement: An Overview and Analysis." In *Self-Regulated Learning and Academic Achievement*, 2nd edition, edited by B. J. Zimmerman and D. H. Schunk, 1–39. New York: Routledge.

Zimmerman, B. J., and M. Martinez-Pons. 1990. "Student Differences in Self Regulated Learning: Relating Grade, Sex, and Giftedness to Self-Efficacy and Strategy Use." *Journal of Educational Psychology* 82: 51–59.

Chapter 3

Using a Readiness Set

FOCUS OF THE CHAPTER

How to develop a Readiness Set to get the student's interest at the onset of a lesson or at the beginning of a new lesson. After the Readiness Set, the teacher plans the lesson to "make sense" and have meaning for the student.

INTRODUCTION

The Readiness Set has three components: the starter (also called a catalyst, hook, or attention getter), the connection of what will be taught to what students know, and the tie-in of the new information to the student's prior knowledge. What does brain research say about getting the student's attention and holding it? Why use a Readiness Set? How does a Readiness Set promote sense and meaning?

Probing Questions

1. How will the teacher get his or her students interested in today's lesson?
2. How will the teacher focus student attention throughout the lesson?
3. What is forward and backward framing, and how can it be used in instructional delivery?
4. How will the student use self-regulation throughout the lesson?

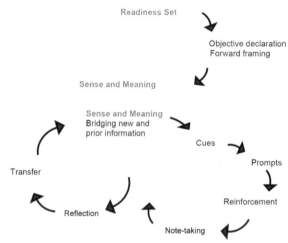

Figure 3.1.

READINESS SET BACKGROUND

Theorists such as John Dewey, Madeline Hunter, and Alfred North White-head focused their scientific learning theories and research on which teacher strategies positively affected and increased the area of student learning in the classroom. It seems that educators today seldom discuss or read Dewey, Hunter, or Whitehead or their work as theorists, and instead turn to the new brain research theories, programs, and innovations presented to them.

Everything Old Is New Again

Pat Wolfe, founder of Mind Matters Inc., observes, in her work, that, quite possibly, the most effective teaching strategies of twenty years ago, such as Hunter and the earlier works of Dewey and Whitehead, are still relevant today because current cognitive and neuroscience research is continually proving the theories of the past to be instrumental in today's world of education.

The current research on the mechanisms of the brain articulates the need for and the promotion of a Readiness Set. Our human brain immediately starts sifting and sorting through all of its sensory input, and simultaneously our brain searches through previously stored information, disseminating new information as potential hooks. A Readiness Set increases the possibility that the brain will search through the right networks and attend to the information that is meaningful for a particular topic or issue.

In order for the brain to fully utilize the potential of the Readiness Set, the level of stress of the task in the classroom must be appropriate. If a task is either too difficult or too easy, the student will have little motivation to continue to the end goal, and it will interfere with efficient learning. More recently, the emphasis is on "productive struggle" so students will be forced to think about the problem presented to them.

Neurons That Fire Together, Wire Together

Today, neuroscientists agree with neurons firing together statement, as they believe that procedural memory is the result of linked circuits or networks of neurons. When circuits and neurons are used repeatedly, they get accustomed to firing together and eventually become hardwired and will fire automatically. Hence the adage that wired-together neurons are neurons that are fired together or, simply stated, "Neurons that fire together wire together." The wiring together comes from connections, which are made, between the new knowledge and prior knowledge.

Neurons Firing Together and the Relationship to Prior Knowledge

Brain research has increased our understanding of why prior knowledge plays an important role in learning as it helps one to better understand how and why the brain learns or doesn't learn. By gaining a scientific understanding of the brain of our learners, teachers can make better decisions about how to structure learning environments and plan effective instructional delivery. Madeline Hunter and other prominent theorists of that time would be ecstatic to know that their early findings are grounded in today's brain research.

READINESS SET

At times, we have all heard a familiar tune and we think to ourselves: "I have heard that song before." The song may bring us back to a place and time that elicits fond memories. It may also bring us unhappy memories. In any event, just remembering the time and place and its relationship to the tune is significant. We may have forgotten over time most of the particulars of what we heard or felt, but once we return to that tune, the emotional memory pours back over us in an overwhelming state.

An experience attached to an emotional event is burned into our memory and, under the right conditions, will surface. Do you remember your favorite high school teacher who always supported you? Do you remember your least favorite high school teacher who made cutting remark? Even though it may be several (or many) years ago, we remember the positive and negative events that have an emotional attachment.

As teachers, we want to plan how information is presented and the content used in the delivery. Most recently in education, there is even less control over content delivered to the students as states have adopted standards to grade levels and a framework for their delivery. Teachers are willing to use the content in the best presentation possible, so that the objectives and principles of the lesson are clear and concise and students can retrieve the information and apply it when necessary in a clear and concise way so that content becomes permanent.

Setting the Stage for Learning

The beginning of a lesson is important as it sets the stage for the information to follow hence the term "Readiness Set." The Readiness Set denotes a way to start a lesson. The Readiness Set sets the stage for learning. Furthermore, this emphasis on setting stage for learning fits precisely with research on the attentional mechanisms of the brain.

In her article "Revisiting Effective Instruction," Pat Wolfe supports the early work done by pioneers in the field, including Hunter's model of Effective Lesson Design, and points out how science researchers have "validated one or another of the practices Hunter espouses" (Wolfe 1998). Brain research has also supported instructional practices addressing the student's emotional level of concern, the role of assessments for task analysis, the promotion of procedural memory and prior learning, and the role of student self-regulation and self-management.

Readiness Set and Research

The Readiness Set has been deemed indispensable by many theorists as enumerated by the research. We have already noted that the Readiness Set is the hook to get the student interest, sets the stage for learning, and focuses the brain to ready itself for the "main attraction." The Readiness Set also adds meaning to the upcoming lesson. Let's use this book as an example.

An Example of a Readiness Set

The purpose of this book is to set the stage for what you wish to learn about self-regulated learning. This book also gained your attention by eliciting a response from you based on your own experiences as both student and teacher. The introduction of the book hooked you into focusing upon what topics were to be presented in each chapter and finally, it provided a framework for you to link prior knowledge to learning and make meaningful connections throughout your learning experience.

Looking Forward or Backward

The Readiness Set is one method to get the student to look forward to the new lesson. Another way is to look "back" or "backward framing."

Restak, in 2006, discussed "Backward Framing" as a concept that addresses the students' prior knowledge to make connections. This concept defined by Restak differs from "forward framing" or telling the student in advance of what they are likely to learn, by using a technique that alters the experience, prior to the student entering into the experience.

The technique is highly regarded in the field of marketing, as this technique alters the consumer's perception and may result in either negative or positive first response. After the marketing strategies are presented, the consumer views the product from a different perspective, and most of the time a change in opinion occurs and it is usually positive.

Framing in communication can be viewed as positive or negative depending on the audience and what kind of information is being presented. The choices that are made are influenced by their creation of a frame. Framing might also be understood as previewing a movie prior to the release of the movie.

If critics post good reviews, moviegoers will go to see the movie expecting a positive experience. How many of us have gone to see a movie based on the "hype" given to it. That is why folks will wait in line to see a movie that is a new release because they heard great things about the movie.

The backward framing is the positive hype that is presented before the person actually sees the movie. The critical component is that positive comments set the stage for a positive experience. In the Readiness Set, the teacher is drawing upon the student's prior experience to set the stage for a positive learning experience.

Information Storage Is Contextual

We remember information in the context in which it is presented. We may forget most of what we heard for a while, but once we hear the information again it will prompt a memory for us. For example, we all have studied the Civil War and Abraham Lincoln. During the course of the study, we are presented information about the assassination of Abraham Lincoln. That information was presented to as an episodic incident: an incident that was presented and stored in our brains, until later when we retrieved it.

Ask someone if they remember the assassinations of Dr. Martin Luther King Jr., or John F. Kennedy (JFK), and most folks will recall studying about these two individuals, as there is meaning and significance attached to their names. Both Dr. King and JFK were connected to a movement or mind-set, and the information was not processed as an episodic event or a single event, but in the context of a bigger frame of reference.

As new information is attached to previous knowledge, the isolated information becomes more meaningful. A link is forged with the new information in one's brain. The teacher can draw upon that information for backward framing when developing a new social studies lesson on assassinations or leaders who stood for a cause. In essence, the teacher is preparing or referring to earlier materials to stimulate the learner.

Using a Sparkler to "Forward Frame"

Teachers can engage students using a Readiness Set in two ways. One, as an introduction, a "sparkler" (forward framing or "sparking" the student's interest in the new material), and as a "catalyst" (backward framing of planting the seed for a positive experience). In both cases, it is to hook into the student's prior knowledge.

Backward or Forward Framing

The Readiness Set can be done using forward or backward framing. Backward framing, as discussed earlier, differs from "forward framing" (telling the students in advance of what they are likely to learn) in that it is a technique used to alter an experience before exposing the experience. Marketers use the technique to alter established memory that includes the viewer's opinion. Positive previews of this will have an impact on the viewer prior to the viewer seeing the movie.

If a movie has a good review after it opens, positive statements are again presented to solidify the previous comments. The backward framing is the "catalyst" used after the movie to get folks to go and see it. The forward framing is the "sparkler" to get folks to go to the movie and see it.

We use forward or backward framing because we remember information in the context in which it was presented as all learning involves emotions. We may forget most of what we heard for a while, but once we hear the information again in an emotional context, it will prompt a memory.

During the course of study about the Civil War and Abraham Lincoln, information was presented as an episodic incident, in that, information was presented at that time and it was stored in the learner's memory.

When information is presented to a movement or mind-set, the information is not processed as an episodic event or a single event, but in the context of a bigger frame of reference. As such, new information is now attached to previous knowledge, and the isolated information becomes more meaningful. The information was linked to a broader context, that is, a movement or mind-set.

FOCUSING STUDENT ATTENTION

One way to focus students and gain their interest is to use props. A prop is something that can be used in creating or enhancing a desired effect. While students are reading a chapter book, "The Cricket in Times Square" (Seiden 1970), a teacher might use a map of Grand Central Station, as a prop for a Readiness Set. The prop will hook the student's interest and serve as a visual aid toward learning.

The next step for the teacher is to isolate the prop in such a way so that a connection between the map of Grand Central Station/Times Square and the chapter book depicting Times Square is made. The teacher may state: "I am showing you a picture. Who can tell me about it?" The teacher waits for the responses from the students that may reflect answers such as "It's a map of Grand Central Station and Times Square."

The teacher continues her questioning until the desired response from the students is given. Then the teacher states, "Correct, this is a picture of Grand Central Station." The teacher continues the questioning. "Has anyone ever been to Grand Central Station? What do you think happens there? Have you ever been to Times Square? Can you tell me what happens at Times Square? What happens at Times Square on New Year's Eve?" The teacher states, "It is a very popular station and it is near Times Square and that is where our chapter book story takes place."

The entire time the teacher is asking questions and soliciting answers from the students, she is referring to the visual aid prop. At this point, the teacher will use a marker to circle the areas on the map that relate to the areas in the chapter book that are the same. The teacher continues her questioning as she works (or has a student identify the areas of New York City). She states, "Have you ever been to New York? Tell me what you liked about New York. Today we are going to read a story about Times Square."

The teacher continues to say, "When we read about a place that is familiar, it rings a bell in your head, so raise your hand if you can share your experience. Today's lesson is about making meaningful connections for you. When we do this together, we learn about each other and we can each gain understanding of our chapters in this fun-filled book!"

Many times, local public libraries have interesting props that can be used for various pieces of literature. A prop can be homemade too. Anything that supports a lesson in some way is a prop. A word, a song, a movie clip, or even a one-liner joke can be a support to a lesson that makes a connection for the student.

Readiness Set versus "Review Time"

Making connections and getting student interest is the desired result for the Readiness Set. A way that a Readiness Set is misused is when it is called "review time." The time that the Readiness Set is supposed to be presented is used instead to review homework, take attendance, pass out papers, or a variety of tasks not related to tying in prior knowledge. The notion is that instruction will begin after the classroom management tasks are completed.

The point, however, is that the time used for a Readiness Set is specific and directed toward activating prior knowledge and not an opportunity to do classroom management tasks. The goal is to provide stimulus that relates in some way to the lesson content: Hook—Connect—Tie. Simply stated, hook the student's interest, connect the new information with the student's prior knowledge, and tie in everything with the lesson.

An Example of a Readiness Set

So let's see what a Readiness Set would look like in a kindergarten lesson plan.

Topic: Patterns
Theme: Patterns All around Me
Overall Objective: I will be able to create four geometric patterns using five shapes.
Objectives: I will be able to correctly identify four geometric shapes and three patterns in nature and everyday life.
Readiness Set: (Teacher will brainstorm with students by using questioning to promote readiness for the lesson and to stimulate prior knowledge—forward framing).
Teacher States: "Who can name some things they saw on the way to school? What shapes were they? Look around the room and name some shapes that you see" (Teacher checks for student learning by finding out what shapes the students made a connection to from the day prior's lesson). This also helps to tie in the student's knowledge. If children cannot name the shape on their own, ask them to "phone a friend" for a possible shape.

Teacher States: "Today we are going to continue our discussion about shapes in the classroom and then talk about shapes outside of the classroom."

Teacher prompts the students by questioning,

"Yesterday we talked about different shapes which included circle, square, triangle, rectangle, and octagon. Can someone give me examples of any one of the shapes?"

"If I ask you what shape the clock is what would you say? What shape is the ceiling tile? What shape is the floor tile? What shape is the fire prevention sign, and one more, what shape is the red stop sign by the door?"

Teacher States: "Since we identified shapes in the classroom, let's think about the shapes outside the classroom. I know a few of you reported that you passed some houses on the way to school."

"Who said they passed Rahim's house? Great, let's close our eyes for a minute and visualize Rahim's house. If you didn't see Rahim's house, then visualize any house that you know about like your own (connections)."

"I am going to get my marker and I am going to ask each one of you to come up to the whiteboard to draw all of the shapes that are in and on Rahim's house!"

"Here we go!" The teacher continues to prompt the students with questions when they get "stuck." The teacher uses a drawing of Rahim's house as her ongoing *prop*.

Examples: "What shape is his house? (Students draw a square.) Did it have a roof? What shape was the roof? (Students draw a triangle.) Now think hard about this one, how about the windows, what shape were they? Who would like to share something they saw and tell us what shape it is?"

Conclusion: The teacher checks for student understanding by evaluating the drawing on the whiteboard, as each child participates and then asks the children to draw their own house on a piece of 8.5 × 11 inch paper and then evaluates the individual progress of each student.

The teacher should remain consistent with the shape objective, but can allow the students to be creative. Within that creativity, it is hoped that the students will be noting that they are creating shapes as they draw.

The above questions and activities help to focus the students' attention (asking questions related to the classroom), tie in the students' frame of reference (looking at shapes on the way to school or tying in a house of a classmate or their own), and tie it all together by reviewing shapes and then identifying them.

Teachers will spend the first few minutes of class, about five to seven minutes, prior to beginning the lesson to develop the Readiness Set. The focus of the above questions and the activities that coincide with the questions will get the student ready for the lesson.

What Does Brain Research Say about a Readiness Set?

Brain research relevant to the Readiness Set includes:

- The review of previous material stimulates prior knowledge. The key to the Readiness Set is to help the brain see relationships.
- Ask questions and have students make predictions. When students make predications, dopamine is released when they are correct. The dopamine rush causes a pleasurable feeling and a pleasurable feeling makes a connection for the child to a positive school climate.
- Ask questions to promote metacognition. The higher levels of Revised Bloom's Taxonomy (RBT) promote metacognition because students are asked to analyze, evaluate, synthesis, and/or create thereby applying factual knowledge.
- Ask students questions related to their frame of reference (their classroom, their home, a friend's home) to help them see relationships.
- Tying the new lesson to the students' school experience ensures that students will have a frame of reference tied to school. They may have different home experiences, but they all come to school and have common experiences in the classroom.
- The Readiness Set creates patterns and relationships, helps to put the lesson in "context," and promotes relevance.
- The use of a prop to gain attention makes the brain connection stronger.
- Research on primacy and regency is addressed as new information is presented at the beginning of the class. This is the principle that the most recently presented items or experiences will most likely be remembered best. If you hear a long list of words, it is more likely that you will remember the words you heard last (at the end of the list) than words that occurred in the middle. This is the regency effect. One will likely remember words at the beginning of the list more than words in the middle, and this is called the primacy effect.

Now that we understand the value of a Readiness Set, the following are examples of Readiness Sets.

TEN EXAMPLES OF READINESS SETS

Here are ten quick and effective strategies that are not only helpful but also easy to implement. As mentioned in the two sample lessons and the research earlier, be sure that you're consistent and hold students accountable for participation. As students become accustomed to the routine, you'll find that an effective Readiness Set will help your students launch into learning, on task and on time!

Ask students to do the following:

1. Circle the home learning (I prefer home learning to homework) questions or problems they would like to discuss. This becomes a discussion point for tying in the previous work with new work. An alternative would be for the students to draft their own questions for when they come to class.
2. Star the homework questions or problems they can explain, and this becomes an *entrance ticket* to the class the next class.
3. Come into class and every person shares *keywords* which he or she has *highlighted* from his or her notes in the previous lesson. He or she can discuss in groups of four keywords and then draft a sentence or two using the keywords.
4. Have a question posed on the board which can be a passage, statement or quotation and ask students to do a *quick write* for 15 seconds on what they know about the question.
5. *Application.* Share with a partner and discuss how the new student learning objective can be applied. Read the objective to the students then ask them to think about an application of what they will be learning.
6. *Making meaning.* Ask students to make meaning of what they will learn. What does today's lesson mean to you? How do you relate to what we will be studying? Based on the information that the teacher hears, tie in the students' frame of reference with the new material.
7. *Focused list.* Create a list of keywords for the students and have the list on the whiteboard and as a handout. Write a message and ask the students to complete the message. Present a problem to the students that will require information from the lesson to solve.
8. *Tie in.* Ask students to complete the sentence: "This makes sense to me because I know x or have experienced x and today's lesson will tie in by. . . ."
9. *Connect.* Complete a brief graphic organizer or a Venn diagram.
10. *Create an "I know list."* Ask students to list what they may already know about the day's lesson.

EXAMPLES OF READINESS SETS FOR LESSON PLANS

Readiness Set for a Science Lesson

How High Is It?

Lesson Objectives

I will learn and be able to justify a tracking device to measure the height of very tall objects such as flagpoles, trees, and telephone poles using triangulation to determine altitude.

I will learn and be able to teach how to measure the elevation angle.

In a subsequent lesson, I will apply the same skills to determine how high a model rocket is launched.

STANDARDS ADDRESSED AND EXPECTATIONS OF STUDENTS

Mathematics

Grade 5 Numbers and Operations:

Solve real-world problems involving the division of unit fractions by non-zero whole numbers and division of whole numbers by unit fractions, for example, by using visual fraction models and equations to represent the problem. *For example, how much chocolate will each person get if three people share 1/2 lb of chocolate equally? How many 1/3-cup servings are in two cups of raisins?*

Strands and Cumulative Progress Indicators:

Building upon knowledge and skills gained in preceding grades, by the end of Grade 12, students will:

A. Numerical Operations

1. Reinforce indicators from previous grade level.
I will be able to measure, record, and use a formula to calculate the altitude.

B. Geometry and Measurement

1. When performing mathematical operations with measured quantities, express answers to reflect the degree of precision and accuracy of the input data.
Objective: I will be able to perform the mathematical operation with accuracy.

C. Patterns and Algebra

1. Apply mathematical models that describe physical phenomena to predict real-world events.
Objective: I will be able to apply the mathematical model to predict the height

of the very tall objects such as flagpoles and tall trees. In a follow-up lesson, I will apply the mathematical model to predict the height of a model rocket when it is launched with an A engine and a B engine.

D. Data Analysis and Probability

    1. Construct and interpret graphs of data to represent inverse and nonlinear relationships, and statistical distributions.

    Objective; I will be able to construct a graph that shows the altitude of the tall objects.

    Mathematics (Common Core State Standards, Grade 4, Geometry). Draw and identify lines and angles, and classify shapes by properties of their lines and angles.

    CCSS.MATH.CONTENT.4.G.A.1. Draw points, lines, line segments, rays, angles (right, acute, obtuse), and perpendicular and parallel lines. Identify these in two-dimensional figures.

    CCSS.MATH.CONTENT.4.G.A.2. Classify two-dimensional figures based on the presence or absence of parallel or perpendicular lines, or the presence or absence of angles of a specified size. Recognize right triangles as a category and identify right triangles.

    CCSS.MATH.CONTENT.4.G.A.3. Recognize a line of symmetry for a two-dimensional figure as a line across the figure such that the figure can be folded along the line into matching parts. Identify line-symmetric figures and draw lines of symmetry.

Readiness Set

Using a *quick write* activity, ask the class: Have you ever wondered how high that _____ is up there? After the quick write, ask students to *pair–share* their answers.

Application. Pair–share with a partner and discuss how the new student learning objective can be applied. Ask the students to think about their answers, share their answers, and then think about another application of what they discussed.

Making meaning. Ask students to make meaning of what they will learn. What does today's lesson mean to you? How do you relate to what we will be studying? To make meaning, students will build a tracker and then track the altitude of a flagpole, trees, and other stationery objects. In future lessons, the student will participate in the building and launching of two different model rockets. The students will track the altitudes of flying model rockets using two different size engines

**Readiness Set for a Workshop on Boys and Girls
Learning Styles**

Read from the book titled *The Minds of Boys* by Michael Gurian, but do not
tell the group the title of this book.

1. *Read aloud the following paragraph:*

"I didn't focus well on what teachers wanted me to do.
I had trouble sitting still for as long as was needed.
I wanted to learn one thing well rather than constantly move between tasks.
I didn't want to read textbook after textbook.
I got bored easily.
I wanted to do my learning, not hear about it.
I was never sure I understood the directions I was given, nor did I succeed
    at accomplishing all of what my teachers demanded.
I often didn't see why I had to be in school anyway."

2. Ask the question:

WHO AM I?

*The answer I was looking for is "it is a male student,
it is a boy!"*

Now we know that the answer is a male, let's talk about the characteristics
we discussed.

I am going to pass out a handout about learning styles, *highlight keywords
from* the handout. They can discuss in groups of four keywords and then draft
a sentence or two using the keywords. Continue to address the group and tell
them that today we are going to talk about the learning styles of boys and
girls. Teacher should say: what were the hints in the paragraph that gave you
the hints? Did the paragraph engage you to think? Continue to ask open-ended
questions in order to direct thinking to the male and female learning styles.

Now that we have hooked the student's interest, the next phase will be to
get the student to participate in the lesson. Student participation is based on
the lesson making sense and having meaning.

The next chapter will answer the question: Why are we learning this?

BIBLIOGRAPHY

Cox, Carol. 2008. "Good for You TV: Using Storyboarding for Health-Related Television Public Service Announcements to Analyze Messages and Influence Positive
Health Choices." *Journal of School Health* 78 (3): 129–186.

Dewey, John. 1897a. *My Pedagogic Creed.* http://www.rjgeib.com/biography/credo/dewey.html.

———. 1897b. "The Psychology of Effort." *Philosophical Review* 6: 43–56.

———. 1910. *How We Think.* Lexington, MA: D. C. Heath.

———. 1913. *Interest and Effort in Education.* Boston, MA: Houghton Mifflin.

———. 1916. *Democracy and Education.* New York: Free Press.

———. 1930. "How Much Freedom in New Schools." *The New Republic* 63: 204–206.

———. 1933. *How We Think: A Restatement of the Relation of Reflective Thinking in the Educative Process.* Boston: D. C. Heath.

———. 1938. *Experience and Education.* New York: Collier Books.

———. 1940. *Education Today.* Westport, CT: Greenwood Press Publishers.

———. 1965. "Education from a Social Viewpoint." *Educational Theory* 15 (3): 73–104.

———. 1969. *The Educational Situation.* New York: The Arno Press.

Hunter, M. 1979. "Teaching Is Decision Making." *Educational Leadership* 37 (1): 62–67.

———. 1982. *Mastery Teaching.* El Segundo, CA: TIP Publications.

Kaufman E. F., J. S. Robinson, K. A. Bellah, C. A. Aviers, P. Haase-Wittler, and L. Martindale. 2008. "Engaging Students with Brain-Based Learning." Atteonline.org.

Kitchel, T., and R. M. Tones. 2008. "Meaning as a Factor of Increasing Retention." Proceeding of 2005. American Association for Agricultural Education, National Research Conferences, San Antonio, Texas.

Pollock, Jane E. 2007. *Improving Student Learning One Teacher at a Time.* Alexandria, VA: Association for Supervision and Curriculum Development.

Robinson, Daniel B., and Doug Gleddie. 2011. "Gym Class with Ed Fizz: Exploring Questionable Pedagogical Practices with Pre-Service Physical Education Teachers." *JOPERD—The Journal of Physical Education, Recreation & Dance* 82 (6): 41–45.

Schulte, Paige Lilley. May–June 2008. "Making Choices: An Exploration of Political Preferences." *Social Education* 72 (4): 10–15.

Wolfe, Pat. 1998. "Revisiting Effective Teaching." *Educational Leadership* 56 (3): 61–64.

Wolfe, Patricia. 2001. *Brain Matters: Translating Research into Classroom Practice.* Alexandria, VA: Association for Supervision and Curriculum Development.

Chapter 4

Developing Sense and Meaning

FOCUS OF THE CHAPTER

Developing sense and making meaning are required if information is to be stored into long-term memory. How do we use cues, prompts, reinforcement, and note-taking to promote making sense and develop meaning for the student? This phase is stage 2 of the Readiness Cycle.

INTRODUCTION

How is making "sense" and promoting "meaning" developed? Why is sense and meaning necessary in the informational stage and for the closing stage? How is sense and meaning developed at each phase of this stage? The various phases in the sense and meaning process will be discussed in this chapter.

Probing Questions

1. What is the role of making sense and having meaning for a lesson?
2. How can I use cues, prompts, and gestures to focus student attention throughout the lesson?
3. What are student "killer questions?"
4. How will I promote reflection to use for student self-regulation?

Why are we studying this? Will we be able to use this information? Will I be able to use this in the real world? These are some of the many questions teachers are asked by students while teachers are presenting lessons. These types of questions send a powerful message to the teacher, which translates into the fact that the student does not see the value, usefulness, or application of the lesson's subject matter and that what is being taught does not make sense to the student.

Additionally, these kinds of questions tell the teacher that the information presented has little or no meaning to the student. We can speculate that the student has not made a connection of the new material to his or her frame of reference. The meaning of the lesson is lost and of no worth to the student.

The Learner's Brain Model Promotes Sense-Making

The Learner's Brain Model believes that the search for meaning is innate. The human brain wants to learn from the time it is created so there is an innate search for meaning. To aid in the search for meaning, teachers should promote "patterning."

Teachers need to create a schema of patternmaking and sense-making to enable students to see the meaning of what they are learning. Patternmaking and pattern seeking is necessary for learners as the process shows connections and relationships. The connections help to develop a "wholeness" or unity of information.

How Does a Teacher Promote Relationships?

The question teachers ask is: "How do I facilitate the learning, so that the students see relationships of the subject matter to his or her own frame of reference? In addition, how will I facilitate a desired outcome, so that this outcome results in sense, meaning, and a positive connection to the brain of the student?"

Ways to Help Students Make Connections

One way to help students connect with their learning or to develop sense and meaning is to use formative assessments. "How Does This Apply" is a useful classroom assessment tool for prompting student applications of learned material. The process begins when the teacher identifies a principle, theory, or generalization for the student or when the student has read about an important principle, theory, or procedure in class.

The objective is to focus the student's attention on what is being learned and prompt the student to connect new ideas to prior knowledge, think creatively, increase the relevance of learned material, and think how the information can be applied.

The task is to answer the question: "How does it apply?" After this process is internalized, the teacher will give the students a 3×5 index card and ask them to develop at least one real-world application for what they have just learned. The process of applying the principle, theory, or concept will help focus the students throughout the lesson, and intrinsically motivate them to seek the relationship between new information and its application.

This process of determining an application of the skill will enable the students to develop meaning from the learning, because they must describe in detail what they learned and how they will apply it now to the real world. The teacher collects all the cards and reads what the students have listed as their descriptions.

The teacher should help the struggling students better understand the relevance of what they were learning by checking for understanding. By providing this auditory commentary, students gain a better understanding of the relationship of the learning to the application and another learning style is used. The student will be able to work with his or her peers to discuss and further brainstorm the descriptions on the "how does this apply?" cards, furthering their understanding.

Pair-Sharing

An alternative way is for the students to work in pairs to share their ideas. This pair-sharing is also very effective for stimulating another learning modality. Discussions with peers that evolves from the "How does this apply" activity promotes metacognition.

The important point to remember for the teacher is that he or she must ensure that feedback is provided and the feedback is immediate. If students hear incorrect application of the concepts, they may tend to remember the incorrect answer, rather than the correct answer. The teacher needs to "re-align" the student's answer.

Realigning Student Answers

Realignment is when one applies the correct stem to an appropriate question. For example, a student states an application of Newton's third law (for every action there is always an opposite and equal reaction) and then gives an example of how it is applicable in the real world. The process begins with the teacher stating what the student stated: "for every action there is an opposite and equal reaction," was Newton's second law and not the third law. The student then hears the teacher's correction and is able to correctly attach the application answer to the correct principle.

How many times have you heard about or witnessed teachers relating an experience that entailed a review of answers on a test and during the review, a student gives an incorrect answer to a question? The astonishing part of this scenario is even though the teachers corrected the answer, to their surprise, when the quiz or test was given, the teachers found that some students still wrote the incorrect answer that they heard in class.

What Do You Know?

Another way to develop meaning for students is to use an assessment called "What do you know?" It is useful because it helps to focus the student's attention to real-world applications of learned lesson materials. It also gives the teacher information regarding prior knowledge of the students. The assessment activity directs the teacher to prepare three open-ended or multiple-choice questions. Students are then instructed to answer the questions that are posed to them.

Based on the information received from the students, teachers can proceed with the lesson. In addition, throughout the lesson the teacher can refer back to questions that he or she posed to the student. The teacher may ask, "What are we learning today? Then the teacher will tie it back to what the student said he or she knows so there is a constant tie-back to the student's prior knowledge and the current lesson.

The teacher may prompt the class by saying: "Remember, the key points that we will be discussing today and how do they apply to the real world?" To promote student engagement, students should work in pairs to determine meaning, usefulness, and application throughout the lesson. This pair–share model encourages brainstorming and connections, which will lead to better learning and application. These questions posed by the teacher can also be used as a "hook" to engage the students and spark an interest into the subject matter.

Focus Student Toward Sense-Making and Developing Meaning

Sense and meaning are two very important considerations for teachers when developing lessons. More importantly, teachers must employ strategies and techniques that will help to focus the student on the task, as well as activate student's prior knowledge and tie in the new information with the old information.

Using Keywords Strategy

One way to do this is to employ a strategy called "Keywords." The strategy involves the teacher listing keywords on the whiteboard, which describes what will be learned (foreshadowing). The teacher references the keywords throughout the lesson, so that the students will be able to connect the key points being discussed to the new learning objective. To be effective, the teacher must refer back to the keywords and/or ask students to discuss among themselves what the keywords mean to them.

Another variation to this technique is to instruct the students to write a definition of three words on one side of the 3 × 5 index card, prior to the beginning of the lesson. After the teacher provides instruction, students may turn the card over and list the definitions of the original words that were originally selected. The students will compare the before and after definitions and evaluate the similarities and differences. The students will then use their cards as an "exit ticket" to leave the classroom.

Keyword Variation

The teacher will review what the students have written on their cards to determine to what degree they understood the concept. A variation of this exercise might be to present this lesson with students working in pairs in order to develop a specific/focused list of keywords that are spoken by the teacher and that they heard throughout the instruction.

To gain students' attention in a fun-filled way the teacher can play a "Jeopardy" type of game using words from the specific/focused list, which were generated by the students. The purpose of the strategy is to promote student engagement.

When a student is involved and engaged to the meaning of a lesson, the student will gain a better understanding of the objective and conceptual value of the subject matter. When the student reflects and evaluates his or her role and position in the lesson, it will create a learning experience that provides sense and meaning to that individual.

Student-Developed Question to Develop Sense and Meaning

Another useful tool that helps promote a student's requirement for sense and meaning of key concepts is to direct the students to develop questions that will be used for a quiz, test, or class discussion. The teacher should encourage students to use Bloom's Revised Taxonomy to promote the use of high and low order types of questions.

Bloom's Taxonomy refers to the domains or classifications of objectives that educators set for students during learning objectives. After the students submit their questions to their teacher, the teacher will be able to determine the thought process of the students, as it relates to the learning objective and the connection to the students' question development.

The teacher gains pertinent information regarding the student's sense of subject importance. Questions which should have been listed by the students and were not allow the teacher insight into the students' thought process regarding what is important to them or not. Furthermore, this allows the teacher to evaluate what change is necessary to differentiate the lesson and meet the needs of the student, in this or subsequent lessons.

Most importantly, this method of lesson delivery encourages students to research the material and decipher it. After the student perceives the level of importance, then, and only then, can the student pragmatically share the information with the teacher.

Did You Use My Question?

The author has seen student-generated question activity performed in a Middle School classroom and the students enjoyed it. On one occasion, a seventh-grade teacher asked the students to develop questions that may be used on a test. During a trial, the students wrote questions and shared the questions in class. The students understood that this sharing was a review for the test.

Once the teacher collected all of the student questions, the teacher used them as a springboard for a classroom discussion the next day. The teacher called upon a student to answer one of the questions. The student responded by stating that she did not know the correct answer to the question. The teacher replied that he was surprised, as the question was personally submitted by her. The student answered: "I didn't think you would use it."

The teacher reminded the students that in the future, any question may be on the test, so they should be mindful of their submissions. The students actually made an excellent point. The moral of the story is that it is one thing to easily make up questions for a test or quiz, but more importantly, the students need to be taught how to link knowledge or information in the form of a question that will make sense to them. The teacher can also use the student generated questions to give her information as to what studets think is important.

Developing Schemas

Making sense of information and organizing it into memory clusters has been referred to a "schema." Early schema theorists (Anderson, Reynolds,

Schallert, and Goltz 1977; Bransford and Franks 1976; Kintsch 1974; Rumelhart and Ortony 1977; Schank and Abelson 1977; Smith 1975; Thorndike and Hayes-Roth 1979) state that learning occurs when one's experiences are related to previously learned knowledge and the students construct their own personal schema.

In order to construct a personal schema, there are three necessary conditions.

- Input: The learner is presented the information.
- Analyze: The learner analyzes the information using his or her frame of reference.
- Create: The learner analyzes the information, synthesizes the information, and creates meaning or develops a schema based on the data input.

In essence it is a flowchart of input-throughput-output. How can input that will yield positive results be created? Let's look at one way.

Elaborate Interrogation

"Elaborate Interrogation" is a method by which the learner "receives" (input stage) or internalizes the presented material. The process of elaborate interrogation involves "asking students to think beyond facts as stated and to construct reasons why the factual relationships make sense" (M. Beard Pressley, ed., in D. J. Hermann, 1992, 82). In a study conducted by Wood, Prissley, and Winne, students were presented with a paragraph containing information about animals:

The Western Spotted Skunk lives in a hole in the ground.
The skunk is usually found in a sandy piece of farmland near crops.
Often, the stock lives alone but families of skunks sometimes stay together.
The skunk mostly eats corn.
The skunk sleeps just about any time accept between 3 o'clock AM and sunrise.
The biggest danger to the skunk is the Great Horned Owl.

Based on two groups of students, a control group and an elaborative interrogation group, the following study was conducted and results noted. In the elaborative interrogation group, the students were asked to read a sentence as if it were a "why" question. For example, why does the Western Spotted Skunk live in a hole in the ground? Or, they could read the sentence as is and then ask "why?" In either case, the student was to question what he or she read.

Students in the control group were asked to read the text then answer a recall or factual question. The students in the elaborative interrogation group, who had to answer the "why" questions, received higher scores on a test (Wood, Prissley, and Winne 1990, 741–48). The three-letter word "why" had a paramount effect that promoted comprehension in reading for the students.

Teachers can also use the elaborative interrogation techniques during their lesson delivery by asking the students answer "why" question posed during the delivery. Students might "tell their neighbors," do a "think-pair-share" activity, or explain the answer to the teacher. In any case, the objective is for the students to justify their answer.

The purpose of questioning ("why") is to help the students understand, that the sentence has meaning, as noted when the control group read the passage about the Western Skunk. Deeper understandings are sought after. Gaining a deeper meaning rather than just reading the passage enables the students to use their own resources and determine why something was done. The purpose of the activity is to develop sense and meaning.

The purpose of the development of sense and meaning is to prepare the student so he or she can pay attention to the material, remember the material, and later apply the information. The key to this phase is to initiate a process to help the student remember or to get ready for the instruction that follows.

THE READINESS PHASE

Now that we know that sense and meaning are required if information is to be stored into long-term memory, the question is: How is "sense" and "meaning" developed? Sense and meaning is also necessary in the informational stage and in the closing stage. Coincidently speaking, sense and meaning

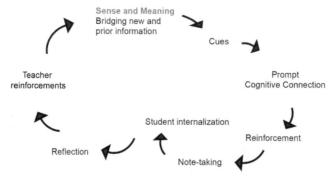

Figure 4.1.

is necessary and important in both stages. Why, then, is sense and meaning developed at each stage? Let's look at the graphic for sense and meaning in the readiness stage.

Readiness, the first stage of instructional delivery, is defined as the preparation of the students toward learning. In order to prepare a student, it is necessary to activate the student's prior knowledge, so that the material being presented will have relevance and meaning to the student.

A cognitive principle is "metacognition" of having the students think about their own thinking. The students need to see a relationship between what they are learning and their prior knowledge; a Readiness Set is used to hook the student's interest, connect the student's prior knowledge, and tie both to the lesson, so the lesson will make sense and have meaning.

Aspects of the Readiness Phase

The concept of Readiness Set is a three-pronged approach: get the student's attention, tie in their prior schemas to the new material, and finally help students make connections. The process is promoted throughout the lesson by the teacher cueing the students or by the teacher scaffolding his or her questions or by the teacher "hooking" the students' attention. Research about effective classroom behavior indicates that cueing and questioning might account for as much as "80 percent of what occurs in a given classroom on a given day" (Marzano 2001, 13; see also Davis and Tinsley 1967; Fillippone 1998).

The Power of Cueing

Cueing is necessary to help focus student's attention to what will be taught. More importantly, cueing helps the student see the relevance to what is being taught, since the student's prior frame of reference is tied to the new knowledge.

The purpose of a cue is to call attention to what the student will be experiencing and/or a way to activate a student's prior knowledge. For example, if students are studying the Vietnam War in social studies class, the teacher may call their attention to the fact that the war was an unpopular one. The teacher may ask the students, what are other examples of unpopular wars?

Since the students discussed various wars prior to the Vietnam War, the cue would be to identify a war previously studied such as the War of 1812. The students would reflect upon similarities between it and the Vietnam War. Cueing questions posed might be: How were they similar? How were they different? During the course of the discussion with students, the teacher can discus the relationships between the wars.

Students may say that both wars were unpopular, and that is the similarity between the Vietnam War and the War of 1812. The "similarity" prompt will help activate the student's prior knowledge and create a relationship tied to the new knowledge. The teacher may delve even further by asking, "Do you remember when we studied wars in general, there was other similar components relating to all wars. Do you remember what they were?" The teacher will wait for answers related to themes such as discontent, a sense of injustice, territorial disputes, and colonization.

Ways to Promote Cueing

Another way to use cues is to write the SLT (objective) on the board and then underline or highlight keywords in the objective. If the objective is: I will be able to correctly distinguish nouns from a list of words, the cue will be for the nouns to be written in a different color ink or different size font.

The purpose of the cue is to distinguish the keyword from the rest of the objective. This technique isolates a key piece of information, thereby making it different and distinct from information around the entire piece of information.

Another suggestion is underlying one word from the "Key Word List," in red ink or changing its size, so that the piece of information stands out among the other information.

When cueing is applied to the objective or Essential Question, the practice has positive implications. Research conducted by Marzano on cueing was reported in several studies: Ross (1988) showed a 16 percent gain; Stone (1983) showed a 27 percent gain; Bloom (1976) showed a 39 percent gain; and Crismore (1985) showed a 23 percent gain (in Marzano 2001, 112).

Using Prompts and Gestures

The teacher may also employ gestures or prompts once the objective is written on the board, as a way to cue the students to keywords. Throughout the lesson, the teacher will point to the keyword. An important aspect of cueing is to ensure that the cues and prompts focus on specific information, which is important and relevant.

The teacher can use gestures, prompts, and cues during class instruction to scaffold student learning. This prompting process helps to focus attention and to develop meaning. Let us examine how the prompting process proceeds.

Prompting a student to focus his or her attention can be done in a variety of ways. Here are some examples of prompting questions:

- After five minutes the teacher will ask the students to share with their neighbor: What was easy, and what was difficult? Students will also be asked to explain their answer so as to begin the process of metacognition.
- After the students complete a cooperative activity, students reflect on what they liked during the activity and what they would do differently. This protocol will lead to robust conversation as students are actually critiquing the lesson and talking about strategies.
- What would you do differently next time you are working in a group?
- Students write in their journals a reflection of the activity answering the question: "Why do you think you were so successful this time and what can you do so you can continue this good work?" Ask this question if the students had been doing poorly in a subject and then improved in their quality of work on a test, report, or project.

Using Voice Prompts and Praise

An additional strategy is the use of voice prompts and praise. This strategy begins after a teacher has taught a lesson and the student is working during the independent instructional phase. During that phase, the teacher will monitor what the students are doing by asking the students to pause and think about or reflect upon what they were studying.

After the student has had time to reflect, the teacher will have an opportunity to dialogue with the student and together they will assess their understanding of the material. If the student is a visual or tactile learner, the teacher may ask the student to show him or her (visual approach) what he or she was working on as opposed to having the student tell (auditory approach) about his or her work. Based on the feedback the teacher receives, a determination will be made by the teacher. The teacher will decide if the student needs to be redirected to review the work or check a stage in the process of doing the work.

To help the students clarify their thinking, the teacher may ask; "How did you arrive at this conclusion?" thereby encouraging the students to explain the process which they used. "How would you defend your answer?" is another question the teacher may ask. The purpose of these questions is to prompt the student to begin the process of metacognition.

To further help the process of metacognition, the teacher may ask probing questions such as "Have you considered . . . ?" The teacher may also involve higher-level questions, so the student can analyze, interpret, synthesize, and form new conclusions. The questioner should develop analytical questions that elicit inferences, analyze supporting or conflicting information, and develop a personal perspective, based on his or her reasoning.

Depending on how the students answer and how the teacher presents questions, the teacher may continue prompting the students and encourage them to dig deeper into the work. The above questions are good examples of probing students to examine their work; however, the student may also be praised for the correct answers. In some cases, even if the praise that is given is verbal, teachers can follow up with a sticker reward.

Often students will have a chart to collect stickers and rewards as a visual aid and external positive reinforcement. The verbal praise should be an observation of what the student is doing and how well that student is doing the task. Remember, vague praise is worthless.

An example of positive praise is, "I see that you have really taken a liking to holding that door open for others. You show the good character trait of helper by doing that so well." This example shows sincere praise. It is not vague but actually targets the exact action of the student. This type of praise quickly connects the task to the positive outcome and emphasizes metacognition within the student's brain function.

Based on the feedback the student receives, the teacher will reevaluate his or her method of instruction and will decide what changes need to take place such as continue the lesson, reteach the skill, or end the instruction and start all over. External and internal reinforcement is important.

Reinforcement will occur during the questioning process, after the student's interests are "hooked" (via the Readiness Set) and/or after the instruction begins as a result of the "cueing."

Positive Praise Leads to Positive Reinforcement

When positive praise is used, it will serve as positive reinforcement on student outcomes. The *Teachers College Record* published a study conducted between 1987 and 2005, which measured instruction using nationally representative samples (*Teachers College Record* 2011). The research revealed that "teachers interactions with students were shown to have a positive association with student outcomes." The key to reinforcement is that the relationships between the teacher and the student must be positive, so that there is trust and acceptance of comments or advice offered by the teacher.

Assuming that teachers understand that a climate of trust in the classroom is important, we then want to ensure that the teacher fully understands how to develop that climate of trust and mutual respect. We want to create an atmosphere for students that engage them in dialogue and make them feel that their opinions are respected.

The Value of Feedback to Create an Atmosphere of Trust

One key way to develop the trust relationship is for the teacher to understand the value of feedback and how feedback is provided to the student. Important considerations for providing feedback, which should be employed by teachers to their students, are as follows:

- Feedback should be tied to standards or rubrics so students know that the feedback is not subjective. Standards-based feedback eliminates allegations of bias or prejudice.
- Feedback should be timely. Timing is important so corrections, adjustments, or changes can be done promptly.
- Feedback should be specific. Vague feedback is no feedback.
- Feedback should promote self-regulation. Encourage students to provide their own feedback so they can begin the process of self-management and self-monitoring.

What Does "Good Job" Mean?

Teachers may often say to the student "good job, well done" or "great" as a way to provide feedback to their students. Although the verbal comments may convey satisfaction on the part of the teacher, they lack clarity as to what is actually meant by "good, well done or great." These words are used all too often and can become repetitive and empty. A student subconsciously reacts to this emptiness, and academic productivity is at risk.

The student likes to hear a positive comment and needs to know that he or she did something that was "good, great" or "well done," but expanding upon these words is necessary. With little effort, the teacher can duplicate these words by recognizing what exactly the student is doing that merited the comment. The teacher's comment must be clearly paired to the desired behavior or the specific action.

To acknowledge a positive situation, the teacher must first observe a specific behavior (i.e., the student is reading a chapter book quietly without disturbing others) and then tell the student exactly what he or she is doing correctly. Once the teacher has noted the specific observable behavior, then the teacher can add positive recognition to the behavior. For example, the teacher may state "X, I see that you are reading your chapter book. You certainly are in great control of yourself and your neighbors must think what a great role model you are for them."

A specific comment will demonstrate to the student immediate clarity, recognition for positive behavior, and set up chapter book expectations for the future. By using this positive reinforcement strategy, the teacher can maintain classroom management with ease. Building a classroom of positive feedback in this fashion will begin to extinguish negative behaviors.

Negative behaviors will become almost extinct because only positive behaviors are recognized. When teachers want to promote a positive behavior, they specify the desired action or task. For example, the teacher may say: "I see the way X is sitting quietly waiting for the next set of directions. Your eyes are focused on me and I like that you are ready." Although the positive behavior is given to one specific student, the whole class observes that student's behavior and the teacher's positive reaction to it.

Talking to one student is internalized by the entire class, and the message to the class is "I am noticed and respected by this teacher" and the behavior is noted. By building the expectations and by giving positive feedback in the correct way, the teacher will find more time for academia and less time spent on disciplining.

Students will be more inclined to display positive behavior than negative behavior, since negative behavior is not recognized in the same way and because people want to create and confirm a positive image of themselves. Negative feedback may make the recipient feel threatened unless they see the value in what they are being told. An educated individual may see that the comment was intended to be constructive as well as informative, and be savvy enough to communicate this to the source. "Constructive feedback" may be seen as "negative," so we usually begin with positive feedback to capture the recipient's attention and involvement and then the focus is on the recipient's behavior. It is also easier to give positive feedback.

Timing Is Important

Additionally, feedback should be given in a timely fashion. Obviously, the more immediate the feedback, the more likely the student will know what is correct. Teachers should be mindful of this concept during their classroom instruction.

Feedback is also important when a student's answer is incorrect. "Realignment" is needed. Attaching a correct answer to the question posed will help the student (and class) make the appropriate association. If the answer and question do not match, the class will hear an incorrect response to a question and make a faulty association. A correction of the error must be made or "re-alignment" is necessary.

For example, in New Jersey, students in grade four study the history of the state, as part of the social studies curriculum. A teacher may peruse a discussion about New Jersey and ask the students to name New Jersey's capital. If a student doesn't know the answer to the question, they may state "Asbury Park" (the correct answer is Trenton, but Asbury Park has notoriety and is known to young adults due to the singer/songwriter Bruce Springsteen who made the city famous).

The teacher needs to correct the student's answer. The teacher should remind the class that the capital of New Jersey is Trenton. The teacher would say, "If we are talking about shore communities, Asbury Park would be one such community and is famous because of Bruce Springsteen. However, capital of New Jersey is Trenton." If the teacher does not correct the student, chances are that when a quiz is given, many students will mention Asbury Park as the capital of New Jersey.

Realignment Strategies

Strategies can be used to promote realignment and self-regulation. Peer editing or group discussions help to promote student self-regulation. While in groups, the students can explain to their peers what they are learning and how the concepts may be applied. They can also use rubrics to evaluate their progress. The discussion with peers allows students to begin to see a broader perspective of the material and to promote metacognition.

While in cooperative groups, another activity that teachers may use is called "I Believe." In this technique, the students are paired and each student defends his or her point of view. The partner then critiques what was heard and has the opportunity to present a response. Each pair discusses the strengths and weaknesses of their point of view. After the discussion, the students attempt to come to consensus. This discussion, dialogue, and discourse promote robust discussions by encouraging students to provide justification for their claims. These activities also help to keep the students interested or hooked.

The Value of Note-Taking

Now that the student's interests are "hooked" and focused on the lesson, students will be encouraged to use note-taking during the lesson. The note-taking will be used to help the students study and focus attention during the lesson. Note-taking and then summarizing the notes is necessary because it helps the students to capture the critical points of a lesson. The notes can be used for metacognition as students can think about what they wrote.

Important factors the teacher needs to consider for effective student note-taking are (1) the pacing of the lesson, which includes both speed and delivery; (2) the level of difficulty of information delivered; and (3) the cues and prompts to be used, which involves verbal and visual signals of emphasis, structure, and relationships.

NOTE-TAKING

What Is Note-Taking?

If note-taking is important, what are the principle functions of note-taking? What strategies are employed? How can note-taking be used to facilitate learning? And more importantly, how can note-taking be taught as an essential skill?

The primary function of note-taking is to record what is being presented, so that the notes can assist at a later date, with study skills. Writing verbatim, what is being said is the least effective way to take notes. Note-taking is a process that the student must learn.

If students record every word that the teacher is saying, it will not allow them to synthesize information into the brain and will not enable them to make sense or develop meaning about what was discussed during the lesson. The working memory of a student will hold information only for about twenty to thirty seconds, then the information is excised unless there is sense and meaning attached to it. When there is no sense and meaning, information will never move from working memory to long-term memory.

Benefits of Note-Taking

Note-taking has great benefits for the learner, for at least two reasons: First, note-taking activates attention mechanisms and engages the learner's cognitive processes of analysis, synthesis, and coding, integrating and transforming verbally received input into a personal and meaningful form. Second, note-taking is seen as beneficial because the recorded notes serve as an external repository of information that permits later revision and review to stimulate recall of information.

Three Generalizations Regarding Note-Taking

The least effective way to take notes is verbatim. Attempting to record everything that is heard or read does not give students a chance to synthesize the information presented. This does not suggest that students should take limited notes; in fact, the more notes the students take, the better. It is important, however, that notes be specific to the learning goals outlined by the teacher. If a student tries to write every word a teachers says, he or she will miss the message. Write what is important.

Note-taking should be a work in progress. Notes should be reviewed, revised, and amended to extend the students' grasp of the content. Students should review their notes for content, clarity, and meaning.

Students should review their notes so the notes become a study guide. A set of clear, well-organized notes can be a powerful tool for test preparation. Students can highlight important words in their notes, summarize their notes, share their notes with study groups. They can select keywords from their notes, think how the notes relate to major concepts and/or Essential Question. In short, students can ask themselves: Why am I learning this?

The Dangers of Round Robin Reading

Every educator knows that problems develop when students focus on every word that is spoken or heard. In the primary grades, teachers observe a lack of comprehension when they engage their students in a technique called Round Robin Reading. In this technique, the student will read of passage, while the rest of the class follows along with their eyes, in their own reader.

After the child reads a passage, the teacher asks the reader what does this passage mean to him or her? It has been my experience that the answer to this question is usually "I don't know." The student is being honest, but the answer may cause an unexpected negative result in the teacher's mind, eliciting a response from the teacher, such as, "what do you mean you don't know, you just finished reading the passage."

The first problem is that the student is not receiving positive feedback from the teacher and will immediately shutdown. Equally important, the student really does not know what he or she read so he or she cannot report. Although this sounds unbelievable, it is true.

The reason for the lack of student comprehension is that the student was probably an inexperienced reader and had to focus on only the words. The student's intention was to "just participate" in the Round Robin Reading assignment. The student could not process the information, as there was too high a demand placed upon the developmental level of the student. The student could only look at each word independently, in order to make no mistakes during their timed reading.

Interesting isn't it? Certainly test it out it in class sometime, but be cognizant of the student's emotions, as this can be a very stressful exercise.

More Note-Taking Strategies

I have deviated from note-taking, but I did want to make a very important point in the previous paragraph. Allow me to continue with more strategies for note-taking.

What strategies can be used to support note-taking? One strategy is pacing. Pacing is an important tool that enables the teacher to help the student process information. If there is a lot of technical information and/or terminology in the lesson, the teacher should be mindful of how fast or slow he or she is delivering the information. This will allow ample time for the student to process what is being presented.

The teacher should set the pace and flow of the information being presented according to the student's readiness and ability. If the student has a strong foundation of knowledge and comprehends the facts, then the teacher should do an informal, on-the-spot evaluation, and possibly hasten the pace of the lesson.

Another way to adjust the pace during note-taking is to pause during the lesson. A pause, or hiatus, during the lesson, helps slow down the pace of the delivery. The teacher can build in "break points" during the lesson, and ask the students to explain what they just learned. This process will set the stage for making connections for the student to the subject matter.

There are also several strategies that can be used to slow the pace of the lesson, which aids note-taking. The teacher can ask the students to pick keywords from the discussion and then share their keywords with the rest of the class. These keywords are heard and remembered by the students.

It is also very important for the teacher to record the words, visually in a chart, as the students recite the keywords out loud. By listening, speaking, and writing the keywords, the teacher is deconstructing the lesson for all of his or her students, resulting in focused attention and memorization.

Another way to pace the lesson is to provide a list of words to the students. While the teacher is instructing the lesson, he or she will be using the keywords. When one of the words is heard within the lecture, the students will be asked to define the word. The class will then engage in a discussion about the definition the classmate proposed. After the class discussion, students will develop a whole "class" definition. This process will slow down the pace of the lesson and help to focus student attention.

For independent assignments, students can review the notes and reflect upon key points, terms, or concepts. The teacher may ask the students to make a list of their keywords and bring it to class the next day. Students can then exchange their list with other students in class and compare what each has written. The students may work in pairs to discuss what was similar and what was different.

Teachers can also develop a game, whereby the class is divided into two teams. A member from team one reads a word from his or her list. A member from team two must define that word. Team two will determine if they have that word on their list. A point is scored for team one if team two does not have the word on their list. In the end, the team with the most points wins the game. During this activity, teachers should take note of the words that are most commonly used that students determined were important.

For example, the teacher may be discussing the Bill of Rights. Keywords reported would be constitution, amendment, fundamental rights, liberties, protection, legislation, ratification, approval, state rights, privacy, search, probable cause, property, and due process. The teacher will informally evaluate the students' performance and understanding of these words, while the students are engaged in a fun-filled team game. If a student does not know the definition, that student may ask a friend on his or her team for support.

Students may have a fun learning experience by playing a game like Jeopardy/Family Feud. The class is divided into two teams. Each team will create their own name (the receiving team and the visiting team). The teacher will write five words under one topic heading and give it to the receiving team. The team will look over the words and think of one clue for each of the words.

The five words will be leveled from easy to hard. The team who has the list of words is going to receive guesses from the visiting team. The visiting team must guess the five words by listening to one clue per word. For every correct answer, they will receive a point. Upon completion of each level, the team will move up the ladder of difficulty. When a mistake is made, the teams will switch roles and the teacher will give five words to the "new" receiving team and the team members will assign one clue to each word.

The game continues until all of the words are discovered and the team with the most points is named the winner. The students may want to use game show terminology like "survey says."

These activities are just a few that can be used to promote retention and help students become familiar with the material. For an extended learning experience and one that will evaluate individual master, a home learning assignment can be given. Students can write a definition of a word that the teacher has provided and use it as an "entrance ticket" to enter classroom the next day. Upon entering the classroom the next day the student will recite what they wrote on their card. The teacher or another student may ask one question of their recording. This enables the teacher to observe, in another format, that the content was mastered.

Remember, the whole purpose of the note-taking, pausing, and reinforcement is to promote long-term retention by giving the student time to process the information. The hope is that the note-taking will lead to long-term retention.

LONG-TERM RETENTION

Educators who want their lessons to be stored in a student's long-term memory, so he or she can retrieve them at a later date must take steps to incorporate sense and meaning into the lesson.

Of the two criteria, meaning has the greater impact on the probability that information will be stored because the information has an emotional connection for the student. We discussed earlier the value of emotions in learning. If the information does not make sense, then the meaning is not clear.

So the question is: How does a teacher strive for meaning? One way is to start the lesson with a Readiness Set, enabling the students to think about an experience, activity, for example, with which they are familiar in order to tie it into the lesson.

The Readiness Set would also help with bridging the new knowledge to the student's frame of reference. Additionally, the use of note-keeping will help with the bridging of information. When a student is encouraged to share his or her note-taking with other students, then the note-taking promotes the process of "making sense" and increases meaning.

When a student is preparing notes in writing, and realizes that these notes will be shared with others in the class, the process of note-taking becomes highly important. The student is motivated to concentrate on how the information will be conveyed and received by others.

A complete system analysis of the process is given below. It begins with the planning stage. The process begins in (1) planning stage/pre-delivery stage. Reflective planning is used in (2) readiness stage, followed by the (3) input stage, and then (4) closure stage.

Lesson Delivery Stage

The purpose of pausing, cueing, and reinforcement is to focus the students' attention. Now that we have the students' interest developed, the class must be made aware of the *lesson objective* and feedback is necessary to complete the task.

FEEDBACK

Both forward framing and backward framing have one thing in common—providing feedback to students. The feedback should be a two-way street, so to speak. It should be reciprocal—from teacher to student and from student to teacher. In fact, students can provide feedback to the teacher (consolidation for closure) on what they learned as well as on their objectives. Student goal setting is a form of providing feedback, to the teacher, as it outlines student expectations. The feedback can be perceived as positive or negative.

Positive feedback, on the other hand, will not be as effective when the student accepts a high grade and an empty, semi-positive comment on a paper such as "great job"; the learner does not know what was positive so they can self-regulate their learning or "good job." This feedback does not provide

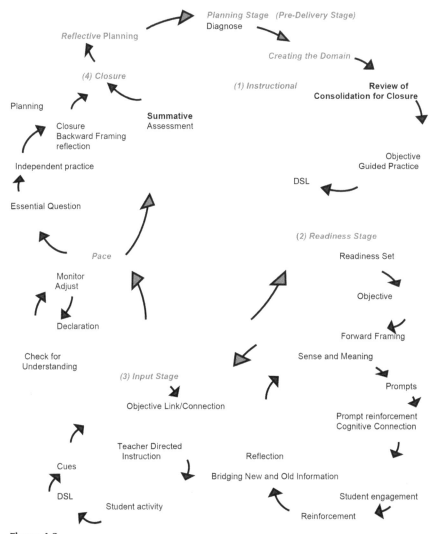

Figure 4.2.

enough specific detail as to what was "good" or "great." Remember, that in the long run, it's just as unproductive not to know why you've done well, as it is not to know why you've done badly.

Here are some tips for providing positive feedback:

- Nonverbal cues are telling, so maintain eye contact with the student.
- Be specific while describing the desired behavior, so the student will know what to replicate in the future.

- Don't mix positive and negative behaviors, as the learner may only hear one and not the other, and it sends a mixed message.
- Praise in public and correct in private.
- Negative feedback, also known as constructive critiques or constructive criticisms, can be used to uncover variables in the student's performance, which the student may not be aware.
- Use constructive critiquing properly to aid the student in avoiding poor performance in the future tasks.
- It's important when using the constructive criticism or constructive critiquing that the teacher is clear.
- Timing is important. In addition, the teacher should relay to the student that he or she is on the "same team" and want to help ensure their success.
- The teacher may also want to consider only using the terminology *constructive*, instead of the words negative or critiquing, as they carry heavy negative connotations and one's brain will *reel into flight or fight*.

Here are tips for providing constructive suggestions (negative feedback):

- "Negative" feedback is usually better when it is given in private so as not to embarrass the student.
- Ask clarifying questions prior to giving specific directions for improvement.
- Ask questions to verify when clarification or feedback is needed. The responses will either verify the need to re-clarify or reteach a lesson or will confirm student understanding.
- Ask questions to promote discussion and statements.
- Evaluate the situation and the student. Anticipate the response you will get when speaking to the student. Ask yourself, "how do I present the information to the student based on what I know about the student?"
- Will the feedback be more manageable for the student coming from his or her peers or from a group discussion?
- Have students set their learning goals and objectives to promote a sense of responsibility for the students.
- To hold students accountable, periodically ask the students to report on the progress of their goals at closure time or during the lesson.
- Question students using low cognitive-type questions, as well as high level of questioning techniques to promote analysis, synthesis, and evaluation.
- The goal of questioning is to promote student achievement in metacognition of the material.
- Use questioning to promote student engagement.

This book focused on the Planning Stage for lesson delivery. In a follow up book, *Activating the Learner's Brain* by Dr. Barbiere, instructional delivery will be discussed.

BIBLIOGRAPHY

Anderson, R. C., R. E. Reynolds, D. L. Schallert, and E. T. Goetz. 1977. "Frameworks for Comprehending Discourse." *American Educational Research Journal* 14: 367–81.

Angelo, T. A., and K. P. Cross. 1993. *Classroom Assessment Techniques: A Handbook for College Teachers*, 2nd edition. San Francisco, CA: Jossey-Bass.

Ashcroft, M. 2006. *Cognition*, 4th edition. Upper Saddle River, NJ: Pearson Prentice Hall.

Black, P., and D. Williams. 1998. "Assessment and Classroom Learning." *Assessment in Education* 5 (1): 70–75.

Bligh, D. 2000. *What's the Use of Lectures?* San Francisco, CA: Jossey Bass.

Bloom, B. S. 1956. *Taxonomy of Educational Objectives*. Boston, MA: Allyn and Bacon.

———. 1976. *Human Characteristics and School Learning*. New York: McGraw-Hill.

Boch, F. 1999. *Pratiques d'écriture et de réécriture à l'université. La prise de notes, entre texte source et texte cible* [*Writing and Rewriting at University: Examples of Note Taking*]. Paris: Presses Universitaires du Septentrion.

Bonwell, C. C., and J. A. Eison. 1991. *Active Learning: Creating Excitement in the Classroom*. Washington, DC: George Washington University.

Branca-Rosoff, S., and J. Doggen. 2003. "Le rôle des indices déclencheurs et inhibiteurs dans les prises de notes des étudiants. Quelques contrastes entre scripteurs 'français' et 'étrangers' [Note-Taking Inhibitory and Releasing Cues by L1 and L2 Students]." *Arob@se* 1–2: 152–66. http://www.arobase.to.

Bransford, J. D., and J. J. Franks. 1976. "Toward a Framework for Understanding Learning." In *The Psychology of Learning and Motivation*, Vol. 10, edited by G. Bower. New York: Academic Press.

Caine, R., and G. Caine. 1997. *Unleashing the Power of Perceptual Change: The Potential of Brain-Based Teaching*. Alexandria, VA: Association for Supervision and Curriculum Development.

Camburn, E. M., and Seing Won Han. 2011. "Two Decades of Generalizable Evidence on U.S. Instruction from National Surveys." *Teachers College Record* 113 (3): 561–610. http://www.tcrecord.org/library ID Number: 16064.

Carrell, Patricia L. 2007. *Notetaking Strategies and Their Relationship to Performance in Listening Comprehension and Communications Assessment Tasks*. Monograph Series, ETS TOEFL, MS—35, ISSN 1550–9012.

Chipongian, L. 2004. *What Is "Brain Based Learning?"* Brainconnection.com.

Crismore, A., ed. 1985. *Landscapes: A State of the Art Assessment of Reading Comprehension Research 1974–1984*. Final Report. Washington, DC: US Department of Education (ED 261–350).

Davis. O. L., and D. Tinsley. 1967. "Cognitive Objectives Revealed by Classroom Questions Asked by Social Studies Teachers and Their Pupils." *Peabody Journal of Education* 44: 21–26.

Davis, W. 2003. *Meaning, Expression, and Thought*. New York: Cambridge University Press.

DeFuze, D., M. Kaplan, and M. A. Deerman. 2001. "Research on Student Note Taking: Implications for Faculty and Graduate Students Instructors" (CRLT Occasional Paper No. 16). Ann Arbor, MI: Center for Research and Learning, University of Michigan.

Dewey, J., and J. A. Boydston. 1965. "Education from a Social Viewpoint." *Educational Theory* 15: 73–104.

Fillippone, M. 1998. *Questioning at the Elementary Level.* Master's thesis., Kean University (ERIC Document Reproduction Service No. ED 417431).

Fuchs, D., and L. S. Fuchs. 1986. "Effects of Systematic Formative Evaluation: A Meta-analysis." *Exceptional Children* 53 (3): 21–29.

Hattie, J. A. 1992. "Measuring the Effects of Schooling." *Australian Journal of Education* 36 (1): 5–13.

Hermann, D. J., H. Weingartner, A. Spearleman, and C. McEvoy, eds. 1992. *Memory Improvement: Implications for Memory Theory.* New York: Springer-Verlag.

Higbee, Kenneth. 1977. *Your Memory: How It Works and How to Improve It.* Englewood Cliffs, NJ: Prentice Hall.

Hunter, R. 2004. *Madeline Hunter's Mastery Teaching: Increasing Instructional Effectiveness in Elementary and Secondary Schools,* updated edition. Thousand Oaks, CA: Corwin Press.

Jackson, Y. 2011. *The Pedagogy of Confidence: In Spring High Intellectual Performance in Urban Schools.* New York: Teachers College Press.

King, S. B., M. King, and W. J. Rothwell. 2001. *The Complete Guide to Training Delivery: A Competency-Based Approach.* New York: AMACOM.

Kintsch, W. 1974. *The Representation of Meaning in Memory.* Hillsdale, NJ: Academic Press.

Kluger, A. N., and A. DeNisi. 1996. "The Effects of Feedback Interventions on Performance. Historical Review: A Meta-Analysis and a Preliminary Feedback Intervention Theory." *Psychological Bulletin* 119: 254–84.

Marzano, R. 1998. *A Theory-Based Meta-Analysis of Research in Instruction.* Alexandria, VA: Association for Supervision and Curriculum Development.

Marzano, R. J., D. J. Pickering, and J. E. Pollock. 2001. *Classroom Instruction That Works: Research-Based Strategies for Increasing Student Achievement.* Alexandria, VA: Association for Supervision and Curriculum Development.

Marzano, R. T., J. S. Marzano, and D. J. Pickering. 2003. *Classroom Management That Works: Research-Based Strategies for Every Teacher.* Alexandria, VA: Association for Supervision and Curriculum Development.

Mcconnell-Cinet, S. 2011. *Gender, Sexuality, and Meaning: Linguistic Practice and Politics.* New York: Oxford University Press.

McREL. 2005. *Classroom Instruction That Works: A Practitioner's Manual for Classroom Instruction That Works.* Research into Practice series. Sandy, UT: School Improvement Network.

Myhill, D., Susan Jones, and Rosemary Hopper. 2006. *Talking, Listening, Learning: Effective Talk in the Primary Classroom.* Maidenhead, UK: Open University Press.

Natriello, G. 1987. "The Impact of Evaluation Process on Students." *Educational Psychologist* 22 (2): 155–75.

Pintrich, P. R., D. A. F. Smith, T. Garcia, and W. J. McKeachie. 1991. *A Manual for the Use of the Motivated Strategies for Learning Questionnaire*. (Tech. Report No. 91-B-004). Ann Arbor: Regents of the University of Michigan, School of Education, National Center for Research to Improve Postsecondary Teaching and Learning.

Rogers, E. M. 1983. *Diffusion of Innovations*, 3rd edition. New York: Free Press.

Ross, J. A. 1988. "Controlling Variables: A Meta-Analysis of Training Studies." *Journal of Educational Research* 58 (4): 405–37.

Rumelhart, D., and A. Ortony. 1977. *The Representation of Knowledge in Memory*. Center for Human Information Processing, Department of Psychology, University of California, San Diego.

Schank, R. C., and R. Abelson. 1977. *Scripts, Plans, Goals, and Understanding*. Hillsdale, NJ: Erlbaum Associates.

Schön, D. A. 1983. *The Reflective Practitioner: How Professionals Think in Action*. New York: Basic Books.

Selden, T. 1960. *The Cricket in Times Square*. Harrisonburg, Virginia: R.R. Donnelley & Sons Company.

Smith, M. C. 1975. "Children's Use of the Multiple Sufficient Cause Schema in Social Perception." *Journal of Personality and Social Psychology* 32(4): 737–47.

Stone, C. L. 1983. "A Meta-Analysis of Advanced Organizer Studies." *Journal of Experimental Education* 51 (7): 405–37.

Thorndike, P. W., and B. Hyes-Roth. 1979. "The Use of Schema in the Acquisition and Transfer of Knowledge." *Cognitive Psychology* 11: 82–106.

Weiner, B. 1972. *Theories of Motivation: From Mechanism to Cognition*. Chicago: Markham.

———. 1974. *Achievement Motivation and Attribution Theory*. Morristown, NJ: General Learning Press.

Weiner, B., I. Frieze, A. Kukla, S. Rest, and R. M. Roenbaum. 1972. "Perceiving the Causes of Success and Failure." In *Attribution: Perceiving the Causes of Behavior*, edited by E. E. Jones, D. E. Kanouse, H. H. Kelley, R. E. Nisbett, S. Valins, and B. Weiner, 95–120. Morristown, NJ: General Learning Press.

Wood, E., M. Prissley, and P. Winne. 1990. "Elaborative Interrogation Effects on Children's Learning of Factual Content." *Journal of Educational Psychology* 82: 741–48.

Appendix A

Checklist for Development of SLT (Objective) and Demonstration of Student Learning (DSL)

	Objective		Indicators	Considerations/Tasks
Alignment	- Objective ties to Essential Question - Objective aligns with Common Core State Standards. - Objective addresses a skill to be assessed by a Criterion Reference Test (CRT) benchmark or curriculum map	☐ ☐ ☐	- High level verbs used - Objective and DSL linked and aligned to standards - Objective is an expectation for skill development and not an activity	- Are Common Core standards "unpacked" in the development of the objective? - Does the objective lead to deeper understanding of the concept? - What is the desired student outcome?
Behavior	- Objective is written using "I" - Objective stresses a student outcome and is not an activity - Lower levels of RBT used to promote factual knowledge which will lead to application (developmental level of skill) or - Higher level verbs used to promote Metacognition - Content and process linked and lead to the development of "dispositions"	☐ ☐ ☐ ☐ ☐	- Begins with "I can, I will" - Clear, specific, measurable so students know what to do - RBT used to develop factual knowledge and base for developing application - Higher level verbs used in the assessment of the skill. - Is the skill needed for the development of a disposition?	- Objective and DSL written in student-friendly terms and appropriate for the age/grade level to promote Self Regulated Learning (SRL) - Factual knowledge necessary to develop creative thinking (Willingham, 2011) to develop skill base for later use. - Assessment (DSL) requires analysis or evaluation to show mastery - "Disposition", i.e., student learns
Condition	- Various strategies planned to deliver the lesson - Delivery of the lesson addresses various student modalities - Technology planned to enhance lesson - Delivery will promote varied grouping practices (large or small groups)	☐ ☐ ☐ ☐	- Instructional strategies used based on student needs. - Variety of learning styles used throughout the lesson - Technology planned for teacher and student use - An outcome of the delivery will lead to flexible grouping	- Varied modalities planned throughout the year. - Students will be able to work at their own pace and self-manage their time. - Technology available for student use and differentiation of lesson - Flexible grouping or use of anchor activities for student who finish early
DSL / Measurement	- Clear connection to objective - High level of Bloom's taxonomy verbs used to assess the learning - Written in student-friendly terms - Measurable – assesses what was taught - Multiple measures of assessment can be used to show mastery - Assessment can be linked to other disciplines - DSL will allow student to create other measures of assessment. - DSLs will lead to "dispositions"	☐ ☐ ☐ ☐ ☐ ☐ ☐	- Objective/DSL congruent - RBT used with emphasis on analyze, evaluate, or create - Students can articulate DSL - Measurement based on rubric or standards - Opportunity for the use of some multiple intelligences - Interdisciplinary approach used for the activities planned. - Student will be able to use multiple measures - DSL mastery can lead to broader use of skill	- Based on student application of information using analysis, interpretation, or creativity - "I can" or "I will show" the teacher - Measurement known to student so student can self-assess throughout lesson - Use of multiple intelligences for product based on student ability - Real-world application promoted to show application of disciplines. - Student expands original assessment to develop other assessments. - Broader applications are expected

Classroom Environment Rubric

Teacher: _____ Room: _____ Grade: _____ Date: _____

	Rubrics	Meaningful Feedback	Routines and Labeling	Student Work Posted
Highly Effective	- Rubrics and exemplars are posted and used - When possible, students have contributed to the development of a rubric - Students refer to rubrics to monitor their progress—self-regulate and self-management	- Feedback is accurate and constructive - Feedback is specific - Feedback is provided in a timely manner - Students can apply the feedback for future learning	- Routines are well established causing no loss of instructional time. - Routines are posted or evident and promotes self regulated learning (SRL). Instructional charts, anchor charts, and labels promote student-directed learning. - Smooth transitions	- Student work is current - Posted work consists of creative student projects - Student work can serve as exemplars of high student expectations - Student work shows pride, attention to detail, and rigor
Effective	- Rubrics are posted, infrequently used. - Students are encouraged to monitor their work—Self Regulate their learning - Students use the rubrics for Self Regulated Learning	- Feedback is accurate - Feedback varies on papers from specific to global - Feedback is provided in a timely manner and for all the papers posted.	- Routines or procedures posted to ensure smooth transitions and effective use of instructional time - Routines are posted or evident and stress high expectations for students - Students transition from one activity to the next smoothly.	- Student work posted varies from high-to-moderate rigor - Student work current but limited in scope - Posted work consists mainly of student projects with no worksheets
Partially Effective	- Some rubrics are posted - Students are aware of the criteria for a specific project or task - Students are aware of the rubric and self-monitor or assess	- Feedback is limited and for one subject - Feedback is generic on some papers and not on other papers - Feedback is provided in a timely manner for most of the papers	- Routines do not appear evident causing loss of instructional time. - Routines are posted or evident by ineffectively applied. - Routines or procedures are posted for class behavior	- Some student work posted - Posted student work has current and non current examples - Posted work a mix of worksheets and student projects
Ineffective	- Rubrics are not posted - Students are not aware of the criteria for grading - Students do not engage in self assessment	- Feedback is very limited and sporadic - Feedback is generic for all papers. Global comments are used "very good" - Feedback is not provided in a timely manner	- Routines do not appear evident causing loss of instructional time. - Routines are not posted or evident - Students are confused by a lack of routines or procedures	- Minimal student work posted - Student work is not current - Posted work consists mainly of worksheets
Student Questions	- *What is the purpose of the rubrics?* - *How often do you use the rubrics?*	- *Does the teacher's feedback challenge you?* - *How does the teacher's feedback help you learn?*	- *Do you know what to do when you are finished with your assignment?* - *How were the routines established?*	- *Why is their student work posted?* - *What do you do if your work is not posted?*

	Student Work	Meaning Feedback	Routines and Labeling	Rubrics
Ratings Highly Effective	⊹ Current ⊹ Creative ⊹ Serve as exemplars	⊹ Accurate ⊹ Specific ⊹ Timely ⊹ Can be applied for future learning	⊹ No loss of instructional time ⊹ Posted ⊹ Smooth transitions	⊹ Posted ⊹ Developed by students ⊹ Used by students
Effective	⊹ Posted with high-to-moderate rigor ⊹ Work current but limited ⊹ Student projects displayed	⊹ Accurate ⊹ Feedback varies ⊹ Timely for many students	⊹ Posted and stress high expectations ⊹ Smooth transitions most of the time ⊹ Some labeling	⊹ Posted, infrequently used ⊹ Students encouraged to use ⊹ Some SRL
Partially Effective	⊹ Some student work posted ⊹ Work not current ⊹ Mostly worksheets	⊹ Limited and sporadic ⊹ Generic or global comments ⊹ Not timely	⊹ Routine not evident or posted ⊹ Loss of instructional time ⊹ Lack of routines	⊹ Some rubrics are posted ⊹ Students are aware of the criteria ⊹ Limited use of rubrics
Ineffective	⊹ Minimal work posted ⊹ Work two months or longer or older ⊹ Posted work mostly worksheets	⊹ Limited and sporadic ⊹ Mostly global comments ⊹ Feedback not timely.	⊹ Not evident ⊹ Loss of instructional time ⊹ Students confused by lack of structure	⊹ Not posted ⊹ Students not aware of rubrics ⊹ No student self-assessment

Differentiated Instruction Rubric

Coaching Suggestions for Differentiated Instruction

Teacher: _____ Room: _____ Grade: _____ Date: _____

	Highly effective	Planning considerations		Notes
Content	Lesson has rigor and requires higher levels of thinking, tied to standards - Frequent checks for understanding employed - Assessments used to monitor and adjust the lesson - Flexible grouping used - Students self-regulate during the lesson	- If the lesson is to be rigorous, what will I use to determine the rigor? - Did I unpack a standard in planning the lesson? - Will higher-order questions be planned to promote critical thinking skills? - Will the lesson build on prior knowledge and lead to creation of a new product or a deeper understanding to the concept taught?	☐	Standards
		- Will there be choice boards, or choice throughout the lesson? - How will I promote application of the skills being taught? - Will the students be given opportunities to analyze their work and share their understanding with their classmates? - How will I know if the students understand what was taught? - Can technology be used to enhance the lesson? - Am I teaching for performance or competency? - If the students are asked "what are they learning, how will they answer?" - Are students demonstrating through their active participation, curiosity, and attention to detail that they value the content's importance? How will I assess their knowledge? - Am I using strategies that promote deep understanding so the content has meaning? - Is my teaching strategy effective in promoting understanding to the extent that students can apply the new knowledge to a variety of real world situations? - Am I allowing students to strengthen their understanding of the content by practicing in a variety of contexts?	☐	Content
		- Am I occasionally withholding information from students to encourage them to think on their own (i.e., Am I asking reflective questions?) - Will I incorporate higher-level questions into the lesson to promote application, analysis, evaluation, and creation? - How will I assess student learning and how often? - Will I use varied methods of assessments? - Will I be using my checks for understanding to modify the pace of my instruction and or the method of my instruction?	☐	Assessments
		- Am I using a variety of strategies to check for understanding throughout all parts of the lesson that will be used to guide my pacing? - How will I determine the pace of the lesson? Will it be student-driven or teacher-driven? - Will I use the environment to promote student self-regulation or self-directed learning so the students can move at their own pace? - Am I planning anchor activities in my lesson for students who finish early? - Am I developing flexible groups based on students' abilities?	☐	Pacing

Process	Variety of learning styles used throughout the lesson - Strategies promote metacognition - Adjustment of lesson made based on feedback and opportunities to practice provided -Variety of instructional strategies used based on student needs	- Will I use Demonstration of Student Learning, Evidence of earnings, Student Assessment of Learning to move students to different skill groups? - Am I planning to teach in a way that provides opportunities for kinesthetic, auditory, and visual learners to succeed and take ownership in their learning (i.e. manipulatives, explicit oral instruction, visual aides)? - Am I using several teaching strategies in one lesson (i.e. whole group direct instruction, small group instruction, project-based learning, and cooperative learning)? - Am I altering my instructional strategies to meet the needs of my students based on their preferred learning styles? - Will I be reflecting on my teaching in order to assess which strategies are more successful than others? - Will I plan to incorporate self-directed learning strategies into the lesson? - Will I use the environment to promote self-regulation? - Will students use written feedback to promote self-regulation? - Will self-regulation strategies be modeled for the students?	☐ ☐ ☐	Learning styles SRL
Product	Formative and summative used - Assessment material posted and used for students to self regulate. - Variety of assessments used based on student choice and tied to the use of standards	- How will I determine student background knowledge? - Will background information gained be used as an assessment that will be used to differentiate the lesson? - Am I planning to use varied types of formative assessments based on different learning styles? - Am I providing students with a choice as to how they will be assessed, that is using student's multiple intelligences to determine the product used to show their understanding of the skill or concept? - How will I use formative assessments to guide my lessons? - Am I planning to use a variety of assessment strategies (i.e. rubrics, checklists, portfolios, oral conversations, projects, presentations, questioning, exit slips etc.)? - Am I providing examples of finished products for students to use as a reference? - Are students given opportunities to self-regulate their learning? - Am I providing students with assessment material that is clearly understood at an early stage in the learning process in order to allow them to self regulate their learning? - When summative assessments are planned, how will I use the information to plan subsequent lessons or activities ?	☐ ☐	Assessments

Interest	- Grouping of students by interest and are flexible - Material connected to student interest - Promote interest beyond classroom - Student suggests choice of project or centers - Products based on student interest and varied use of MI	- - Are students demonstrating through their active participation, curiosity, and attention to detail that they value the content's importance? - Am I drawing on the connections students can make between the content and real life? - Am I taking into consideration the likes and dislikes of my students when designing my lesson plans? - Am I developing conceptual understanding through artful scaffolding and connecting with students' interests? - Are students contributing to extending the content by explaining concepts to their classmates? - Am I using expressive spoken and written language? - Am I finding and embracing opportunities to extend students' vocabularies, both within the discipline and for more general use? - Am I explaining content clearly, using metaphors and analogies to bring content to life? - Is there evidence of student initiation of inquiry and student contributions to the exploration of important content?	☐	- Interests
	- Are student interests identified via multiple intelligences?	- Have I identified student's interests or preferences using a multiple intelligence inventory? - Will interest centers be developed using multiple intelligences, that is a center for verbal linguistic, interpersonal? - Are students aware of their primary and secondary multiple intelligences and can select a center based on their interest of develop a product as evidence of learning the skill or concept?	☐	Multiple intelligences
Readiness	- Assessments determine grouping - Curriculum modified based on student levels - Flexible grouping used based on student interest and abilities	- Am I collecting data, analyzing it, and using it to drive my instruction? - Am I formulating groups based on assessment data in order to better meet the needs of my students? - Am I taking into consideration the readiness of my students when forming groups? - Am I developing modified assignments according to students' abilities? - Am I modifying lessons according students' abilities? - Will I work with small groups of students who demonstrate a lack of understanding or a misconception about the content? If so, what will the other students do?	☐	Assessment

Dispositions "Look fors"	Highly Effective	Disposition	Look "fors"	Questions
Content "Look fors" Standards-based, inter-disciplinary, rigorous, student-centered, authentic	- Tiered activities - Independent activities - Interdisciplinary lesson with higher levels of application -Problem-based learning promoted to show deep understanding of concepts and application. - Will students promote their own learning?	Rigor Standards-based Authentic learning Student-centered	- Lesson tied to standards - More than one discipline presented. - Application of facts to promote student competency - Student metacognition	-Is the essential question, student learning target (objective) and activities tied to learning or an activity? - Are interdisciplinary activities planned to show relationships? - Will the factual information presented be applied? Is it Performance or Competency that is asked? - Will students see relationships of the material and be able to think about applying the information?
Process "Look fors" Structured, dynamic, monitored and adjusted based on feedback, promotes Self-Regulated Learning (SRL)	- Students move at their own pace and self-manage their time. - Student can select from Anchor activities or other resources. - Strategies in place to plan and execute compacting the lesson, that is student learning contracts, independent study, SRL - Student activities planned using multiple intelligence.	Lesson structure Lesson delivery Student activity Variety in delivery	- Lesson planned to progress for whole group to small group. - Individual needs addressed via different starting points _How does the lesson address student variety ? Will multiple intelligences be addressed?	- How will time be managed to move the lesson at an appropriate pace? - How will I plan to compact the lesson? - After the lesson is begun, how will I address students learning at a different pace? - What plans are in place to address students who complete the assignment early? -Will multiple intelligences be used for the production of student products?
Product "Look fors" Summative, diverse, MI used, shows what students Know	- Will students apply the information using analysis, interpretation, or creativity? - Use of multiple intelligences for product based on student ability - Real-world application promoted	- Teacher - Student products	- Will students apply the skills? - Will students be able to use their various intelligences to create products?	- How will students show they know, understand, and can apply information? How will I know that the students understand the skills? - Will students have the option to use their multiple intelligence to produce a product?
Interest Student involvement Activities, student connections, self regulation	- Instruction based on student interest to promote student involvement - Activities student centered and based on individual interests. - Specific, frequent reference to student interest.	- Student interests	Student interest is high Students are actively interested in the lesson and engaged in the lesson	- Do I know my student's interests? If I do will I plan activities based on their interests? - Will I plan for the use of interest centers in the lesson?
Readiness Student skill levels. grouping, assessments to determine levels	- Teacher uses assessments to determine grouping of students - Students engage in SRL – constitutionally and environmentally - Resources available and students encouraged to use them	- Student Prior know-ledge planned	- Student readiness planned to compact the lesson. - Student readiness used initially then lesson is adjusted based in student	- An readiness set is planned to tie student prior knowledge and activate student interest. - After an introductory activity, i.e., readiness set, Do Now, the lesson will flow based on student readiness and interest.

Index

Note: Page numbers in italics indicate figures.

affective domain, 37
Alzheimer's disease, 26
attention. *See* student attention

backward framing, 53, 54–55
behavior, 36; questions to ask when
   considering, 36–37
Bloom's Taxonomy, 38, 69, 70
brain bandwagon, 3–4; early childhood
   education, 4
brain cells, 4
brain research, 2; early educational
   experiences, 10–11; instructional
   delivery and, 16; IQ, 10
Brooks-Gunn, Jeanne, 11
Bush, George H. W., 3, 16

classroom environment, 41–44;
   finding meaning and purpose in, 6;
   twenty-first-century learning, 41–42
Classroom Instruction That Works
   (Marzano, Pickering, and
   Pollock), 35
cognitive domain, 37
communication: framing in, 53
compliance, 25

condition, 36; questions to ask when
   considering, 37
constructive feedback, 78, 86. *See also*
   negative feedback
cooperative groups, 79
cueing: power of, 73–74; promoting, 74

"Decade of the Brain," 3, 16
Democracy and Education (Dewey), 10
developing sense and meaning. *See*
   sense and meaning, development of
Dewey, John, 9–10, 50
Diamond, Marion, 5, 10
DOL (domains of learning), 36, 37–39;
   student-friendly, 39; writing,
   important considerations, 38

early childhood education, 4; federal
   legislation and, 11
effective school research, 20–22
Einstein, Albert, 2
elaborate interrogation, 71–72
emotional environment, 22; for sense
   and meaning, 27
emotional intelligence, 12
emotions, 11–12

About the Author

Dr. Mario C. Barbiere has administrative experience at all district levels and has also taught college classes as an associate professor. He has extensive work experience in school turnaround beginning with serving as Network Turnaround Officer (NTO) for two inner-city schools that had been low performing. Working with the principal and teachers, both schools doubled their test scores in one year and became higher-achieving schools. After that, Dr. Barbiere was executive director for Regional Achievement Center, Region 5, which was created to work with low-performing schools or schools with an achievement gap. Under the Every Student Succeed Act, the Regional Achievement Centers were identified as Comprehensive Support and Improvement Teams and Dr. Barbiere was the regional executive director.

His doctoral studies were in brain research and lesson design. The research developed interest in instructional delivery and student self-regulation.

Having the opportunity to work in a variety of schools, Dr. Barbiere is passionate about teaching and student empowerment so students are empowered and self-dependent and not teacher- or school-dependent.

Lightning Source UK Ltd.
Milton Keynes UK
UKHW01f0539160618

324228UK00001B/27/P